Biologics and Biology-Based Regenerative Treatment Approaches in Periodontics

Editors

ALPDOGAN KANTARCI
ANDREAS STAVROPOULOS
ANTON SCULEAN

DENTAL CLINICS OF NORTH AMERICA

www.dental.theclinics.com

January 2022 • Volume 66 • Number 1

ELSEVIER

1600 John F. Kennedy Boulevard • Suite 1800 • Philadelphia, Pennsylvania, 19103-2899

http://www.dental.theclinics.com

DENTAL CLINICS OF NORTH AMERICA Volume 66, Number 1
January 2022 ISSN 0011-8532, ISBN: 978-0-323-83530-5

Editor: John Vassallo; j.vassallo@elsevier.com
Developmental Editor: Ann Gielou M. Posedio

Dental Clinics of North America (ISSN 0011-8532) is published quarterly by Elsevier Inc., 360 Park Avenue South, New York, NY 10010-1710. Months of issue are January, April, July, and October. Business and Editorial Offices: 1600 John F. Kennedy Boulevard, Suite 1800, Philadelphia, PA 19103-2899. Periodicals postage paid at New York, NY and additional mailing offices. Subscription prices are $323.00 per year (domestic individuals), $854.00 per year (domestic institutions), $100.00 per year (domestic students/residents), $377.00 per year (Canadian individuals), $863.00 per year (Canadian institutions), $100.00 per year (Canadian students/residents) $441.00 per year (international individuals), $863.00 per year (international institutions), and $200.00 per year (international students/residents). International air speed delivery is included in all *Clinics* subscription prices. All prices are subject to change without notice. **POSTMASTER:** Send address changes to *Dental Clinics of North America*, Elsevier Health Sciences Division, Subscription Customer Service, 3251 Riverport Lane, Maryland Heights, MO 63043. **Customer Service (orders, claims, online, change of address): Elsevier Health Sciences Division, Subscription Customer Service, 3251 Riverport Lane, Maryland Heights, MO 63043. Tel: 1-800-654-2452 (U.S. and Canada). Fax: 314-447-8029. E-mail: journalscustomerservice-usa@elsevier.com (for print support); journalsonlinesupport-usa@elsevier.com (for online support).**

Reprints. For copies of 100 or more, of articles in this publication, please contact the Commercial Reprints Department, Elsevier Inc., 360 Park Avenue South, New York, NY 10010-1710. Tel.: 212-633-3874; Fax: 212-633-3820; E-mail: reprints@elsevier.com.

The Dental Clinics of North America is covered in *MEDLINE/PubMed (Index Medicus), Current Contents/Clinical Medicine, ISI/BIOMED* and *Clinahl.*

Contributors

EDITORS

ALPDOGAN KANTARCI, DDS, PhD
Senior Member of Staff/Professor, The Forsyth Institute, Cambridge, Massachusetts, USA

ANDREAS STAVROPOULOS, DDS, PhD, Dr. Odont.
Professor, Department of Periodontology, Faculty of Odontology, University of Malmö, Sweden; Division of Conservative Dentistry and Periodontology, University Clinic of Dentistry, Medical University of Vienna, Vienna, Austria

ANTON SCULEAN, DMD, MS, PhD
Professor, Department of Periodontology, University of Bern, Bern, Switzerland

AUTHORS

NICOLE ARWEILER, DDS, PhD
Department of Periodontology and Peri-Implant Diseases, Philipps University of Marburg, Marburg, Germany

MARK BARTOLD, BDS, BScDent(Hons), PhD, DDSc, FRACDS(Perio)
School of Dentistry, The University of Queensland, Brisbane, Queensland, Australia

FAREEHA BATOOL, PhD
INSERM (French National Institute of Health and Medical Research), UMR 1260, Regenerative Nanomedicine, Fédération de Médecine Translationnelle de Strasbourg (FMTS), CRBS, Université de Strasbourg, Faculté de Chirurgie-dentaire, Strasbourg, France

NADIA BENKIRANE-JESSEL, PhD
INSERM (French National Institute of Health and Medical Research), UMR 1260, Regenerative Nanomedicine, Fédération de Médecine Translationnelle de Strasbourg (FMTS), CRBS, Strasbourg, France

KRISTINA BERTL, DDS, MSc, MBA, PhD
Associate Professor, Department of Periodontology, Faculty of Odontology, University of Malmö, Sweden; Division of Oral Surgery, University Clinic of Dentistry, Medical University of Vienna, Austria

NIDIA CASTRO DOS SANTOS, DDS, MSc, PhD
Assistant Professor, Department of Periodontology and Oral Implantology, Dental Research Division, Guarulhos University, Guarulhos, São Paulo, Brazil

RALUCA COSGAREA, PhD, DDS, PD
Department of Periodontology, Operative and Preventive Dentistry, University of Bonn, Bonn, Germany; Department of Periodontology and Peri-Implant Diseases, Philipps

University of Marburg, Marburg, Germany; Department of Prosthetic Dentistry, University Iuliu Hatieganu Cluj-Napoca, Cluj-Napoca, Romania

MAGDA FERES, DDS, MSc, DMSc
Dean for Dental Research and Graduate Students, Professor, Department of Periodontology and Oral Implantology, Dental Research Division, Guarulhos University, Guarulhos, São Paulo, Brazil

LUCIENE C. FIGUEIREDO, DDS, MSc, PhD
Professor, Department of Periodontology and Oral Implantology, Dental Research Division, Guarulhos University, Guarulhos, São Paulo, Brazil

MERVI GÜRSOY, DDS, PhD
Adjunct Professor, Department of Periodontology, Institute of Dentistry, University of Turku, Turku, Finland

ULVI KAHRAMAN GÜRSOY, DDS, PhD
Associate Professor, Department of Periodontology, Institute of Dentistry, University of Turku, Turku, Finland

PIERRE-YVES GEGOUT, DDS, MSc
INSERM (French National Institute of Health and Medical Research), UMR 1260, Regenerative Nanomedicine, Fédération de Médecine Translationnelle de Strasbourg (FMTS), CRBS, Université de Strasbourg, Faculté de Chirurgie-dentaire, Pôle de médecine et chirurgie bucco-dentaire, Hôpitaux Universitaires de Strasbourg, Dental Faculty, Periodontology, Strasbourg, France

HATICE HASTURK, DDS, PhD
Senior Member of the Staff, Department of Applied Oral Sciences, Director, Center for Clinical and Translational Research, The Forsyth Institute, Cambridge, Massachusetts, USA

OLIVIER HUCK, DDS, PhD
Professor, INSERM (French National Institute of Health and Medical Research), UMR 1260, Regenerative Nanomedicine, Fédération de Médecine Translationnelle de Strasbourg (FMTS), CRBS, Université de Strasbourg, Faculté de Chirurgie-dentaire, Pôle de médecine et chirurgie bucco-dentaire, Hôpitaux Universitaires de Strasbourg, Dental Faculty, Periodontology, Strasbourg, France

SASO IVANOVSKI, BDSc, BDentSt, MDSc(Perio), PhD
School of Dentistry, The University of Queensland, Brisbane, Queensland, Australia

EIJA KÖNÖNEN, DDS, PhD
Professor, Department of Periodontology, Institute of Dentistry, University of Turku, Turku, Finland

ALPDOGAN KANTARCI, DDS, PhD
Senior Member of Staff/Professor, The Forsyth Institute, Cambridge, Massachusetts, USA

KAMAL MUSTAFA, DDS, PhD
Professor, Department of Clinical Dentistry, Faculty of Medicine - Tissue Engineering Group, University of Bergen, Bergen, Norway

HAYRIYE ÖZÇELIK, PhD
INSERM (French National Institute of Health and Medical Research), UMR 1260,
Regenerative Nanomedicine, Fédération de Médecine Translationnelle de Strasbourg
(FMTS), CRBS, Strasbourg, France

GIORGIO PAGNI, DDS, MS
Department of Biomedical, Surgical and Dental Sciences, University of Milan, Foundation
IRCCS Ca' Granda Policlinic, Milan, Italy

CATHERINE PETIT, DDS, MSc
Associate Professor, INSERM (French National Institute of Health and Medical Research),
UMR 1260, Regenerative Nanomedicine, Fédération de Médecine Translationnelle de
Strasbourg (FMTS), CRBS, Université de Strasbourg, Faculté de Chirurgie-dentaire, Pôle
de médecine et chirurgie bucco-dentaire, Hôpitaux Universitaires de Strasbourg, Dental
Faculty, Periodontology, Strasbourg, France

GIULIO RASPERINI, DDS
Department of Biomedical, Surgical and Dental Sciences, University of Milan, Foundation
IRCCS Ca' Granda Policlinic, Milan, Italy

BELEN RETAMAL-VALDES, DDS, MSc, PhD
Assistant Professor, Department of Periodontology and Oral Implantology, Dental
Research Division, Guarulhos University, Guarulhos, São Paulo, Brazil

ANTON SCULEAN, DMD, MS, PhD
Professor, Department of Periodontology, University of Bern, Bern, Switzerland

SIDDHARTH SHANBHAG, DDS, PhD
Department of Clinical Dentistry, Faculty of Medicine - Tissue Engineering Group,
University of Bergen, Department of Immunology and Transfusion Medicine, Haukeland
University Hospital, Bergen, Norway

JAMIL AWAD SHIBLI, DDS, MSc, PhD
Director of Oral Implantology Program, Professor, Department of Periodontology and Oral
Implantology, Dental Research Division, Guarulhos University, Guarulhos, São Paulo,
Brazil

ANDREAS STAVROPOULOS, DDS, PhD, Dr. Odont.
Professor, Department of Periodontology, Faculty of Odontology, University of Malmö,
Sweden; Division of Conservative Dentistry and Periodontology, University Clinic of
Dentistry, Medical University of Vienna, Vienna, Austria

CÉLINE STUTZ, PharmD, MSc
INSERM (French National Institute of Health and Medical Research), UMR 1260,
Regenerative Nanomedicine, Fédération de Médecine Translationnelle de Strasbourg
(FMTS), CRBS, Strasbourg, France

LORENZO TAVELLI, DDS, MS
Department of Periodontics, University of Michigan School of Dentistry, Ann Arbor,
Michigan, USA; Department of Oral Medicine, Infection, and Immunity, Division of
Periodontology, Harvard School of Dental Medicine, Boston, USA

SHUNTARO YAMADA, DDS, MSc
Department of Clinical Dentistry, Faculty of Medicine - Tissue Engineering Group,
University of Bergen, Bergen, Norway

Contents

> The ultimate goal of periodontal therapy is homeostatic regeneration of lost attachment of alveolar bone and gingival connective tissue to the exposed root surfaces with a fully functional and healthy periodontal ligament that is covered with a healthy epithelium. This goal needs a complete understanding of the biological mechanisms inherent to healing and inflammatory processes.

> Periodontitis is a multifactorial inflammatory condition associated with an oral microbiome dysbiosis that results in gingival inflammation and clinical attachment loss. Periodontal therapies are based on scaling and root planing to disturb the bacterial biofilm mechanically and remove calculus and contaminated cementum. Research does not support the use of root modifiers for decontamination and biomodification of periodontally affected root surfaces. Standardized clinical trials in large populations, assessing biological and patient-reported outcome measures, are necessary to evaluate candidate biomaterials for decontamination and biomodification of periodontally affected root surfaces.

> Technological innovations in cellular and molecular aspects of tissue engineering – scaffolds, stem cells and 3D printed tissues – have been dramatically increased in the last decade. However, regenerative treatment still has challenges in translation to clinic. This is partly due to failure of addressing an essential element of wound healing, inflammation. It is now well-recognized that inflammation is an active process. This paradigm shift opened up a new avenue of therapeutic approaches called "host-modulation." Host-modulation therapies capable of modulating inflammatory response at multiple levels and mimicking the natural sequence of wound healing offer a new direction and promising clinical translation.

Successful periodontal regeneration requires the hierarchical reorganization of multiple tissues including periodontal ligament, cementum, alveolar bone, and gingiva. The limitation of conventional regenerative therapies has been attracting research interest in tissue engineering-based periodontal therapies where progenitor cells, scaffolds, and bioactive molecules are delivered. Scaffolds offer not only structural support but also provide geometrical clue to guide cell fate. Additionally, functionalization improves bioactive properties to the scaffold. Various scaffold designs have been proposed for periodontal regeneration. These include the fabrication of biomimetic periodontal extracellular matrix, multiphasic scaffolds with tissue-specific layers, and personalized 3D printed scaffolds. This review summarizes the basic concept as well as the recent advancement of scaffold designing and fabrication for periodontal regeneration and provides an insight of future clinical translation.

Current periodontal treatments aim to control bacterial infection and decrease inflammation. To optimize contemporary conventional treatments that present limitations owing to an inability to reach the lesion site, new methods are based on nanomedicine. Nanomedecine allows delivery of host-modulatory drugs or antibacterial molecules at the lesion site in an optimal concentration with decreased toxicity and risk of systemic side effects. Chitosan and polylactic-co-glycolic acid-loaded nanoparticles, carbon quantum dots, and mesoporous silicates open new perspectives in periodontitis management. The potential therapeutic impact of the main nanocarriers is discussed.

The ultimate goal in periodontal therapy is the complete re-establishment of the lost tissues. Dental researchers and clinicians are continuously working to develop current therapeutic techniques and technologies that can regenerate damaged periodontal tissues. Predicting the outcome of the treatment is a challenging endeavor, because a variety of local and systemic variables can affect the success of the applied regenerative therapy. To real-time monitor the biological changes during periodontitis or after periodontal treatment, various biomarkers have been studied in periodontology. This article discusses the available evidence on the use of biomarkers in the detection of periodontal regeneration.

Biologics and Biology-Based Regenerative Treatment Approaches in Periodontics

DENTAL CLINICS OF NORTH AMERICA

SERIES OF RELATED INTEREST

Atlas of the Oral and Maxillofacial Surgery Clinics
http://www.oralmaxsurgeryatlas.theclinics.com

Oral and Maxillofacial Surgery Clinics
http://www.oralmaxsurgery.theclinics.com

THE CLINICS ARE AVAILABLE ONLINE!
Access your subscription at:
www.theclinics.com

Introduction

Vision of Regenerative Periodontology

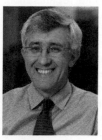
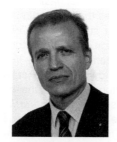
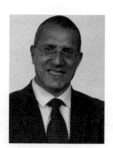

Alpdogan Kantarci,
DDS, PhD

Andreas Stavropoulos,
DDS, PhD, Dr. Odont.
Editors

Anton Sculean,
DMD, MS, PhD

Retaining teeth in natural occlusion and function, being esthetically and harmonically integrated with oral-facial esthetics, is the ultimate goal of dentistry. Implants led to a paradigm shift in restorative dentistry and provided excellent options in replacing missing teeth.[1] Still, considering the challenges with the relatively frequently appearing mechanical and biological complications at implants, these should only be offered when the natural teeth are missing or cannot be retained. Regenerative periodontics has revolutionized the clinical practice and can deliver predictable solutions for restoring the lost tissue integrity around the teeth, provided proper case and treatment selection and execution, empowering dentists to successfully manage periodontal disease and keep their patients' teeth in their mouths. To achieve both hard and soft tissue regeneration is not an easy task and requires an in-depth understanding of biology, anatomy, physiology, and pathology. Teeth are exposed to an external environment, flooded with one of the most diverse microbiomes in the human body, and under the continuous functional forces, and thus present a unique challenge that the other medical professionals do not experience.[2] Periodontal tissue regeneration not only builds what is lost but also promises a functional unit that is resilient to microbial and physical insults.

We are living in exciting times when science and research are more translatable and practically within reach for clinicians. This volume was planned before the Covid-19 pandemic of 2020 to 2021. As in many other fields in medicine, the pandemic was a challenging time for dentists. Many of us worked through and survived this unprecedented phase in the history of human civilization. As being truly frontline workers everywhere in the world, we adapted and learned how to provide our services to our patients. We also became more aware of what we can do as dental professionals to restore our patients' health. The pandemic also provided us with innovation that has

Dent Clin N Am 66 (2022) xi–xiii
https://doi.org/10.1016/j.cden.2021.08.002

never been experienced in human history. Furthermore, resources of the scientific world combined with a global urge to fight against the pandemic have truly translated scientific research to every corner of the globe through vaccines. Such scientific advancements will be incorporated in understanding the mechanisms and developing of treatment strategies for many diseases, including periodontitis.

The timing of this volume is critical. Although we are building on our understanding of periodontal regenerative medicine, we incorporate the most recent technologies. The journey starts with an overview of the biological basis of periodontal regeneration. We then cover one of the most critical issues that determine the success of regenerative approaches: decontamination of root surfaces and keeping the environment infection-free. Next, we focus on inflammation as a modulator of periodontal regeneration and how we can take advantage of recent innovations in the resolution of inflammation as a regenerative strategy. This is followed by an excellent article on stem cells and their potential in periodontal regeneration that paves the way for the next 2 articles on clinical approaches for hard and soft tissue regeneration. We then move on to the long-term outcomes following regenerative techniques and on how these approaches can improve long-term tooth prognosis. The final 2 articles are focused on emerging nanomedicine concepts in periodontal regeneration and the use of biomarkers in the prediction and prognosis of clinical procedures.

Overall, this volume is intended to bring the experts in this field to look into future applications and technological advances. It is not our intention to replace excellent and comprehensive reviews and consensus reports.[3–12] However, our goal is to pave the way for an updated, but also simplified, understanding of innovation in periodontal practice to deliver our promise of the retention of patient's teeth.

Alpdogan Kantarci, DDS, PhD
Forsyth Institute
245 First Street
Cambridge, MA 02142, USA

Andreas Stavropoulos, DDS, PhD, Dr. Odont.
University of Malmo
Carl Gustafs väg 34
Malmö 214 21, Sweden

Anton Sculean, DMD, MS, PhD
University of Bern
Freiburgstrasse 7
Bern 3010, Switzerland

E-mail addresses:
akantarci@forsyth.org (A. Kantarci)
andreas.stavropoulos@mau.se (A. Stavropoulos)
anton.sculean@zmk.unibe.ch (A. Sculean)

REFERENCES

1. Lang NP. Oral implants: the paradigm shift in restorative dentistry. J Dent Res 2019;98(12):1287–93.

2. Joseph S, Curtis MA. Microbial transitions from health to disease. Periodontol 2000 2021;86(1):201–9.

3. Giannobile WV, Jung RE, Schwarz F, Groups of the 2nd Osteology Foundation Consensus Meeting. Evidence-based knowledge on the aesthetics and

maintenance of peri-implant soft tissues: Osteology Foundation Consensus Report Part 1-Effects of soft tissue augmentation procedures on the maintenance of peri-implant soft tissue health. Clin Oral Implants Res 2018;29(Suppl 15):7–10.

4. Murakami S, Bartold M, Meyle J, et al. Group C. Consensus paper. Periodontal regeneration–fact or fiction? J Int Acad Periodontol 2015;17(1 Suppl):54–6.

5. Scheyer ET, Sanz M, Dibart S, et al. Periodontal soft tissue non-root coverage procedures: a consensus report from the AAP Regeneration Workshop. J Periodontol 2015;86(2 Suppl):S73–6.

6. Reddy MS, Aichelmann-Reidy ME, Avila-Ortiz G, et al. Periodontal regeneration - furcation defects: a consensus report from the AAP Regeneration Workshop. J Periodontol 2015;86(2 Suppl):S131–3.

7. Cochran DL, Cobb CM, Bashutski JD, et al. Emerging regenerative approaches for periodontal reconstruction: a consensus report from the AAP Regeneration Workshop. J Periodontol 2015;86(2 Suppl):S153–6.

8. Reynolds MA, Kao RT, Camargo PM, et al. Periodontal regeneration - intrabony defects: a consensus report from the AAP Regeneration Workshop. J Periodontol 2015;86(2 Suppl):S105–7.

9. Tatakis DN, Chambrone L, Allen EP, et al. Periodontal soft tissue root coverage procedures: a consensus report from the AAP Regeneration Workshop. J Periodontol 2015;86(2 Suppl):S52–5.

10. Kao RT, Nares S, Reynolds MA. Periodontal regeneration - intrabony defects: a systematic review from the AAP Regeneration Workshop. J Periodontol 2015; 86(2 Suppl):S77–104.

11. Sanz M, Simion M, Working Group 3 of the European Workshop on Periodontology. Surgical techniques on periodontal plastic surgery and soft tissue regeneration: consensus report of Group 3 of the 10th European Workshop on Periodontology. J Clin Periodontol 2014;41(Suppl 15):S92–7.

12. Hammerle CH, Giannobile WV, Working Group 1 of the European Workshop on Periodontology. Biology of soft tissue wound healing and regeneration–consensus report of Group 1 of the 10th European Workshop on Periodontology. J Clin Periodontol 2014;41(Suppl 15):S1–5.

Biological Basis of Periodontal Regeneration

Alpdogan Kantarci, DDS, PhD*

KEYWORDS

- Periodontal regeneration • Biologics • Tissue engineering

KEY POINTS

- Understanding the current status of the biological basis of periodontal regeneration will enable the adoption of emerging strategies in clinical practice for retaining natural teeth.
- Developing therapeutic approaches that will take advantage of tissue biology and physiology.
- Predicting the outcomes of periodontal regenerative procedures.

INTRODUCTION

One of the oldest debates in periodontal therapy has been the regeneration of the lost tissues due to the disease process. The basis for this ongoing discussion is the complexity of disease mechanisms of initiation, progression, and resolution. Being an open interface between the soft and the hard tissues of a highly active and functional unit involved in mastication and exposed to microbial elements and environmental factors makes the periodontium one of the most complex biological structures in nature. The infection and inflammatory processes affecting the homeostatic stability of the periodontal tissues lead to its destruction and involves the failure of several cellular and molecular mechanisms of defense. Consequently, substantial resources and efforts are focused on understanding periodontal disease pathogenesis. Restoring periodontal structures and regeneration of the lost soft and hard tissues must be based on the exact same pathways that destroy tissue components. It would not be too ambitious to refer to "periodontal regeneration" as more complex than soft tissue-only regeneration (eg, skin) or hard tissue-only regeneration (eg, bone) because periodontal regeneration involves all of these in a highly contaminated and open wound and a highly functional environment in the oral cavity.

The first detailed experimental evidence for periodontal regeneration can be traced to a publication in 1934 in which Stones[1] presented compelling histologic data supporting that root cementum can regenerate in nonhuman primates. In this seminal paper, various critical observations relevant to the modern understanding of periodontal

Forsyth Institute, 245 First Street, Cambridge, MA 02142, USA
* Corresponding author.
E-mail address: akantarci@forsyth.org

Dent Clin N Am 66 (2022) 1–9
https://doi.org/10.1016/j.cden.2021.08.001
dental.theclinics.com

regeneration were made. First, epithelial cells were shown to repopulate the entire root surfaces denuded of cementum, producing a weak and unstable attachment with dentin, easily separated from the root surface. Second, regeneration of cementum was demonstrated to be possible due to new cementoblasts lining the healing tissues, whereas alveolar bone has the capacity to regenerate. Finally, space was identified as critical to regeneration. This work also showed that pathologic disruption of the periodontal attachment could be reversed and restored by the remaining cells of the periodontium. These observations were confirmed in dog studies in the 1950s[2-4] and collectively demonstrated that periodontal regeneration was feasible, differentiating the reattachment from new attachment with conclusive evidence.

During the next 2 decades, cellular origins of periodontal regeneration were identified.[5] Melcher[5] proposed the critical cells in the periodontium that could be responsible for the outcomes for treatment. Meanwhile, several surgical techniques have been introduced for periodontal regeneration. The advancements for the past 40 years of research since the early 1980s allowed periodontology to be a pioneer in regenerative medicine. Owing the extensive research at the basic science and translational levels, we now appreciate a better understanding of the processes underlying the clinical therapeutic choices (**Fig. 1**). This article focuses on the biological mechanisms underlying periodontal regeneration, identifying key molecular and cellular processes and noncellular elements of the periodontal regenerative process.

REPAIR OR REGENERATION: CONCEPTUAL TO BIOLOGICAL WOUND HEALING

In the absence of any regenerative techniques, periodontal surgery led to a wound healing that was predominantly a repair.[6,7] Early studies were based on the histologic analyses of human models and demonstrated 3 histopathological levels of corona apically positioned layers: epithelium, connective tissue, and cementum-bone interface. Given the limited amount of cementum-bone interface, which was defined as "periodontal attachment," these studies suggested that periodontal surgical techniques without any regenerative strategy are limited in their capacity to restore lost tissues. This observation led to a major paradigm shift in periodontology. Studies in the 1980s demonstrated periodontal regeneration as a feasible outcome in periodontal treatment using innovative techniques.[8-17] Most importantly, however, regenerative

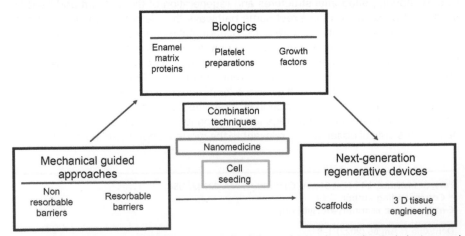

Fig. 1. Periodontal regeneration as a process that combines the mechanical devices and biologics.

approaches led to a deeper understanding of biology-based treatment strategies to restore periodontal tissues to their levels before the disease.

Every form of wound healing includes regeneration. The distinction between "repair" and "regeneration" is conceptual rather than biological. Repair has been used to refer to an incomplete or lack of regeneration where cellular elements populate the wound area depending on their proliferation rates and activities after an injury inflicted by periodontal surgery. Therefore, cells with higher multiplication, growth, and proliferation capacity would be the first to arrive at the injury site. Not surprisingly, similar to the other wound models elsewhere in mammals, epithelial cells originating from the gingiva have the highest migration and proliferation capacity. Thus, wound healing by repair starts with epithelial cells covering the wound area. This stage should be seen as a defensive action to protect the site from being infected by excluding the injury site from the environment. On the other hand, it also prevents an actual attachment of the hard tissues and complete regeneration of periodontal ligament on the exposed root surfaces. Therefore, periodontal epithelization has been perceived as a protective but limiting step in regeneration, leading to disruption of homeostatic wound healing during the repair.

Based on these fundamental observations, "guiding" periodontal regeneration has been introduced as a clinical technique.[18–21] Guided regeneration refers to intentionally directing the specific cells to where they should be located to restore tissues. To this end, it differs from the random/natural repair process after surgical wounding, where regeneration is limited and unpredictable. Many guided strategies included the prevention of epithelization on the root surfaces. Physical prevention of epithelialization along the denuded root surface was thought to allow dental and periodontal cell sources to proliferate and populate, leading to a new attachment.[22] The first generation of guided periodontal regeneration involved the use of nonresorbable barriers, which required removal. The need for a second surgery was overcome by introducing resorbable barriers, which provided varying degrees of resorption times and sources to the clinicians. The operator's case selection and technical skills were critical in the success of guided periodontal regenerative approaches,[23,24] which became the gold standard in periodontal therapy. In the absence of an epithelial seal around the tooth, it has also become apparent that the spatiotemporal reconstruction of periodontal ligament and hard tissues with an optimal attachment of alveolar bone to cementum through fibers was not always predictable.

Precision and timing are critical for periodontal regeneration. Periodontal wound healing is not a linear process. All cell types are present and functional at the same time. Regeneration is the outcome of an orchestrated proliferation, differentiation, synthetic activity, and apoptosis of individual cell lineages.[25]

CELLULAR REGULATION OF PERIODONTAL REGENERATION

Early research suggested the involvement of epithelial cells, gingival fibroblasts, periodontal ligament fibroblasts, cementoblasts, osteoblasts, osteoclasts, and osteocytes in the healing after periodontal treatment. In addition to these primary cells with structural roles, endothelial cells, immune cells, and neuronal cells are critical in regulating periodontal regeneration. Wound healing was initially thought to follow similar stages of development of dentoalveolar and dentogingival structures. However, we now know that there are profound differences in the origin of cells involved in the healing of damaged tissues of the periodontium.[26,27] For example, the oral epithelium replaces the odontogenic epithelium in forming the junctional epithelium at the dentogingival junction. Gingival and periodontal ligament fibroblasts become the primary stromal cells during wound healing, replacing the dental follicle. Progenitor stem cells in the periodontal ligament and mesenchymal stem cells from the endosteal spaces differentiate into cementoblasts, fibroblasts, and osteoblasts, replacing the dental follicle and dental papilla.[28] These observations suggested 2 critical points: (1) wound healing is different in adult periodontal and dental tissues than the neonate and (2) cells regulating wound healing in the adult need to be identified to predict periodontal regeneration.

On the other hand, identifying prenatal and postnatal processes during the tooth eruption and formation of the periodontium led to the first completely biological regenerative strategy in periodontal therapy. Enamel matrix proteins were introduced as mediators of periodontal regeneration owing to their multifaceted functions. While increasing epithelial cell attachment for optimal wound closure, these embryonic proteins stimulate fibroblastic proliferation and activity of cells in the gingiva and periodontal ligament. Most importantly, they regulate the endothelial function by chemotactic stimulation of endothelial cells, which is essential for homeostatic wound healing. The effect of enamel matrix proteins is not equal on all cell types; proliferation of periodontal fibroblasts is favored over gingival fibroblasts and epithelial cells, which allows periodontal attachment to take place before the denuded root surfaces could be populated by the gingival connective tissue cells and epithelium. Simultaneously, osteogenic cell proliferation is stimulated, preparing an osseous wall for the new attachment to connect. Mechanistically, enamel matrix proteins were shown to stimulate various transcriptional factors, growth factors, and mediators involved in osteoblastic, cementoblastic, and odontoblastic cell function.[29] These studies demonstrated the role of biological mediators as proregenerative strategies in the absence of physical barriers. Thus, enamel matrix proteins and other growth factors that have been introduced for periodontal regeneration represent the third generation of guided regenerative approaches.

Several growth factors have been tested for periodontal regeneration. Recombinant human platelet-derived growth factor, insulinlike growth factor, bone morphogenetic proteins, fibroblast growth factor, growth/differentiation factor are among those that have shown promising clinical results with strong preclinical and in vitro supporting data.[30,31] Platelet preparations offer packaged growth factors and other components of wound healing (eg, lipoxins) involved in the regenerative process.[32–39] These preparations can be used in combination with other regenerative procedures and continue to evolve.

Biologics offer more directed stimulation of cells and molecules to be recruited to the site of the surgical injury. However, the issue of spatiotemporal guiding of periodontal regeneration has still not been addressed. Current regenerative strategies involve the controlled release of growth factors and other biologically active molecules using various scaffolds and other tissue-engineered constructs that offer a prolonged delivery while maintaining the wound space.[40,41] Another regenerative approach uses nanoparticles that are loaded with biologics. In addition, gene therapy presents many opportunities for regenerative medicine, including periodontal regeneration.[42] These "smart" regenerative techniques allow the recruitment of different cell types and molecules needed for tissue regeneration in the periodontium and, when used in combination, will address the programmed regeneration at the site of injury.

At the cellular level, stem cells in the periodontium have received substantial attention as critical regulators of types of cells involved in the regenerative process. As periodontal ligament stem cells are multipotent progenitor cells, they can proliferate and differentiate into required cell types of the periodontium. This observation was groundbreaking because it demonstrated that periodontal tissues did have the capacity to regenerate if the stem cells could be mobilized and directed toward a predictable periodontal regeneration.[43] Indeed, in response to various growth factors, adhesion molecules, and extracellular matrix components, progenitor multipotent periodontal ligament stem cells can differentiate into precementoblasts, prefibroblasts, and preosteoblasts and subsequently commit to the mature cells of these lineages (ie, cementoblasts, fibroblasts, osteoblasts).

Under the optimal conditions and in the absence of any inflammation or infection, periodontal regeneration can be seen as an orchestration of these cell types along the exposed root surfaces. Inflammation, however, is an impactful determinant of the outcomes of healing along with the immunologic factors. Systemic causes of inflammation, such as diabetes and cardiovascular diseases, result in an impaired regenerative process.

MOLECULAR BASIS OF WOUND HEALING AND PERIODONTAL REGENERATION

In healthy tissues, gingival connective tissue presents similar characteristics to the skin.[44–46] Collagen and noncollagenous matrix (eg, proteoglycans, fibronectin, elastin) are produced by gingival fibroblasts at varying degrees depending on the topographic and functional features. Oral mucosal wound healing follows 4 phases: (1) hemostasis, (2) inflammation, (3) new tissue formation and cell proliferation, and (4) maturation and matrix remodeling. The hemostasis phase involves coagulation, enrichment of platelet and other hematological elements in coagulum, and fibrin meshwork with coagulum to generate "provisional extracellular matrix." This phase is followed by the inflammatory recruitment of immune cells and other cellular components to regulate tissue turnover. Neutrophils and monocytes arrive in the wound area; macrophages are differentiated from monocytic precursors into proinflammatory M1 phenotype or proresolutive M2 phenotype. The transition of the inflammatory phase to the proliferative phase is the most critical step and requires an infection-free environment. During this transition, granulation tissue derived from the periodontal ligament induces epithelial cells to form a keratinized masticatory gingiva. Granulation tissue is a healing vasculature and fibroblast-rich extracellular matrix regulating endothelial cell recruitment for new capillary vessels. At this step, fibroblasts are recruited from wound edges and pericytes. Epithelial-mesenchymal transition involves the formation of epithelium from keratinocytes, whereas the soft connective tissue determines the characteristics of the overlaying oral epithelium. In return, oral epithelium determines connective tissue healing. Therefore, epithelial-mesenchymal communication is a central event in wound healing and regeneration. Although there is an overlap between epithelial and connective tissue regeneration, there is also a gap in timing. Typically, epithelial healing takes 7 to 14 days following nonsurgical and surgical periodontal therapy. Functional stability between the denuded root and soft tissue is achieved approximately 14 days after surgery. Therefore, the timing of these events is crucial for optimal healing.

The periodontal ligament is dissimilar to other tissues in the mammalian body. It is primarily a connective tissue and therefore contains collagen types I and III as the major proteins with Sharpey fibers attaching to the cementum. Another unique tissue is the periodontium is the root cementum. Although structurally similar to other hard tissues, alveolar bone and cementum are uniquely attached through predominantly collagen fibers. All these structures are vascularized through the vessels in the gingiva and periodontal ligament.

Degradation of the extracellular matrices can occur through various pathways, including activation of matrix metalloproteinases, the release of reactive oxygen species cytokine release, and prostaglandin synthesis cell activation. Upon injury, 3 types of wound healing may occur, all of which are regulated by inflammation. The ideal healing is by full regeneration after a complete resolution of inflammation. However, when the inflammation cannot be resolved and becomes chronic because of the inability to eliminate the injurious agent or insufficient coping by the immunoinflammatory process, 2 scenarios may occur: (1) tissue destruction and (2) fibrosis. Both tissue responses also represent healing but not an ideal regeneration. Thus, in almost all types of healing, there will be areas of destruction and fibrotic changes. At the same time, minimal regenerative sites emphasize the role of inflammation as a master regulator of healing. Clinically, however, the 3 distinct models are recognized as pathologic conditions (chronic inflammation associated with periodontal tissue destruction or fibrotic expansion of periodontal tissues) or regenerative healing.

In addition to the inflammation as a process, several critical molecular events and mediators are actively involved after the injury; these include growth factors, cytokines, chemokines, lymphokines, and various tissue factors released from inflammatory cells and damaged tissue. These molecules trigger a cascade of signaling reactions as a prelude to their action and lead to the production of further molecular mediators. Although these markers of inflammation were thought to be detrimental, they were also involved in wound healing. Therefore, inflammatory resolution and reprogramming are key for regenerative wound healing. Likewise, extracellular matrix proteins can be used as regenerative biologics when combined with scaffolds.[47]

SUMMARY

Periodontal regenerative medicine is a predictable procedure when the underlying biological process is understood. Many surgical techniques and materials have been used to deliver this clinical outcome. Bone grafts, growth factor preparations, platelet derivatives and preparations, scaffolds, nanoparticle-based delivery systems, stem cells, and gene therapies are currently being tested for the spatiotemporal predictability of periodontal regeneration.[48] Sufficient and convincing evidence is accumulating to support several applications such as growth factors.[49] Meanwhile, the inflammatory resolution is being tested as a tool to allow the cells of the periodontium to repopulate on the exposed root surfaces.[50] Reprogramming the stemness of periodontal ligament stem cells under inflammatory conditions may offer a wider capability for regenerative periodontal therapy in clinical practice. Cells may become irrelevant when we can obtain and deliver the small extracellular vesicles of exosomes of stem cells for periodontal regeneration.[51] The field has moved to a more biological-based understanding of periodontal regeneration to address the mechanism of healing. Recruitment of specific cell types to the site of injury is feasible. A customized strategy[48] with vascularization of the regenerated tissue and innervation of the newly formed structures fully integrated with the native tissues and mechanoresponsive[52] will focus on future studies to accomplish the ultimate goal of maintainable regeneration.

CLINICS CARE POINTS

- Although dental implants offer excellent solutions for restoring edentulism, the goal of periodontal therapy is to restore and retain natural teeth as a functional and healthy unit. Periodontal regeneration is feasible and predictable, offering a wide variety of treatment options to clinicians.

DISCLOSURE

Nothing to disclose.

REFERENCES

1. Stones HH. The reaction and regeneration of cementum in various pathological conditions: (section of odontology). Proc R Soc Med 1934;27:728–44.
2. Linghorne WJ, O'Connell DC. Studies in the regeneration and reattachment of supporting structures of the teeth; soft tissue reattachment. J Dent Res 1950; 29:419–28.
3. Linghorne WJ, O'Connell DC. Studies in the regeneration and reattachment of supporting structures of the teeth. II. Regeneration of alveolar process. J Dent Res 1951;30:604–14.
4. Linghorne WJ. Studies in the reattachment and regeneration of the supporting structures of the teeth. IV. Regeneration in epithelized pockets following the organization of a blood clot. J Dent Res 1957;36:4–12.
5. Melcher AH. On the repair potential of periodontal tissues. J Periodontol 1976;47: 256–60.
6. Orban B. Gingivectomy vs. conservative treatment of periodontal diseases. J South Calif State Dent Assoc 1948;15:15–7.
7. Stahl SS. Repair or regeneration following periodontal therapy? J Clin Periodontol 1979;6:389–96.
8. Nyman S, Karring T, Lindhe J, et al. Healing following implantation of periodontitis-affected roots into gingival connective tissue. J Clin Periodontol 1980;7:394–401.
9. Karring T, Nyman S, Lindhe J. Healing following implantation of periodontitis affected roots into bone tissue. J Clin Periodontol 1980;7:96–105.
10. Nyman S, Lindhe J, Karring T. Healing following surgical treatment and root demineralization in monkeys with periodontal disease. J Clin Periodontol 1981; 8:249–58.
11. Nyman S, Gottlow J, Karring T, et al. The regenerative potential of the periodontal ligament. An experimental study in the monkey. J Clin Periodontol 1982;9:257–65.
12. Nyman S, Lindhe J, Karring T, et al. New attachment following surgical treatment of human periodontal disease. J Clin Periodontol 1982;9:290–6.
13. Gottlow J, Nyman S, Karring T, et al. New attachment formation as the result of controlled tissue regeneration. J Clin Periodontol 1984;11:494–503.
14. Karring T, Isidor F, Nyman S, et al. New attachment formation on citric acid and non-citric acid treated roots. J Periodontal Res 1984;19:666–9.
15. Lindhe J, Nyman S, Karring T. Connective tissue reattachment as related to presence or absence of alveolar bone. J Clin Periodontol 1984;11:33–40.
16. Isidor F, Karring T, Nyman S, et al. New attachment-reattachment following reconstructive periodontal surgery. J Clin Periodontol 1985;12:728–35.
17. Karring T, Isidor F, Nyman S, et al. New attachment formation on teeth with a reduced but healthy periodontal ligament. J Clin Periodontol 1985;12:51–60.
18. Gottlow J, Nyman S, Lindhe J, et al. New attachment formation in the human periodontium by guided tissue regeneration. Case reports. J Clin Periodontol 1986; 13:604–16.
19. Nyman S, Gottlow J, Lindhe J, et al. New attachment formation by guided tissue regeneration. J Periodontal Res 1987;22:252–4.

20. Pontoriero R, Lindhe J, Nyman S, et al. Guided tissue regeneration in degree II furcation-involved mandibular molars. A clinical study. J Clin Periodontol 1988; 15:247–54.
21. Pontoriero R, Lindhe J, Nyman S, et al. Guided tissue regeneration in the treatment of furcation defects in mandibular molars. A clinical study of degree III involvements. J Clin Periodontol 1989;16:170–4.
22. Caton JG, DeFuria EL, Polson AM, et al. Periodontal regeneration via selective cell repopulation. J Periodontol 1987;58:546–52.
23. Polson AM, Caton J. Factors influencing periodontal repair and regeneration. J Periodontol 1982;53:617–25.
24. Burkhardt R, Lang NP. Fundamental principles in periodontal plastic surgery and mucosal augmentation–a narrative review. J Clin Periodontol 2014;41(Suppl 15): S98–107.
25. Susin C, Fiorini T, Lee J, et al. Wound healing following surgical and regenerative periodontal therapy. Periodontology 2000 2015;68:83–98.
26. Aukhil I, Iglhaut J. Periodontal ligament cell kinetics following experimental regenerative procedures. J Clin Periodontol 1988;15:374–82.
27. Iglhaut J, Aukhil I, Simpson DM, et al. Progenitor cell kinetics during guided tissue regeneration in experimental periodontal wounds. J Periodontal Res 1988;23: 107–17.
28. Pitaru S, McCulloch CA, Narayanan SA. Cellular origins and differentiation control mechanisms during periodontal development and wound healing. J Periodontal Res 1994;29:81–94.
29. Bosshardt DD. Biological mediators and periodontal regeneration: a review of enamel matrix proteins at the cellular and molecular levels. J Clin Periodontol 2008;35:87–105.
30. Kaigler D, Avila G, Wisner-Lynch L, et al. Platelet-derived growth factor applications in periodontal and peri-implant bone regeneration. Expert Opin Biol Ther 2011;11:375–85.
31. Stavropoulos A, Wikesjo UM. Growth and differentiation factors for periodontal regeneration: a review on factors with clinical testing. J Periodontal Res 2012; 47:545–53.
32. Miron RJ, Moraschini V, Fujioka-Kobayashi M, et al. Use of platelet-rich fibrin for the treatment of periodontal intrabony defects: a systematic review and meta-analysis. Clin Oral Investig 2021;25:2461–78.
33. Ozcan E, Saygun I, Kantarci A, et al. The effects of a novel non-invasive application of platelet-rich fibrin on periodontal clinical parameters and gingival crevicular fluid transforming growth factor-beta and collagen-1 levels: a randomized controlled clinical study. J Periodontol 2020. [Epub ahead of print].
34. Miron RJ, Zucchelli G, Pikos MA, et al. Use of platelet-rich fibrin in regenerative dentistry: a systematic review. Clin Oral Investig 2017;21:1913–27.
35. Eren G, Kantarci A, Sculean A, et al. Vascularization after treatment of gingival recession defects with platelet-rich fibrin or connective tissue graft. Clin Oral Investig 2016;20:2045–53.
36. Oncu E, Bayram B, Kantarci A, et al. Positive effect of platelet rich fibrin on osseointegration. Med Oral Patol Oral Cir Bucal 2016;21:e601–7.
37. Tunali M, Ozdemir H, Kucukodaci Z, et al. A novel platelet concentrate: titanium-prepared platelet-rich fibrin. Biomed Res Int 2014;2014:209548.
38. Yassibag-Berkman Z, Tuncer O, Subasioglu T, et al. Combined use of platelet-rich plasma and bone grafting with or without guided tissue regeneration in the treatment of anterior interproximal defects. J Periodontol 2007;78:801–9.

39. El-Sharkawy H, Kantarci A, Deady J, et al. Platelet-rich plasma: growth factors and pro- and anti-inflammatory properties. J Periodontol 2007;78:661–9.
40. Vaquette C, Pilipchuk SP, Bartold PM, et al. Tissue engineered constructs for periodontal regeneration: current status and future perspectives. Adv Healthc Mater 2018;7:e1800457.
41. Tavelli L, McGuire MK, Zucchelli G, et al. Biologics-based regenerative technologies for periodontal soft tissue engineering. J Periodontol 2020;91:147–54.
42. Lin Z, Rios HF, Cochran DL. Emerging regenerative approaches for periodontal reconstruction: a systematic review from the AAP Regeneration Workshop. J Periodontol 2015;86:S134–52.
43. Ivanovski S, Gronthos S, Shi S, et al. Stem cells in the periodontal ligament. Oral Dis 2006;12:358–63.
44. Bartold PM, Narayanan AS. Molecular and cell biology of healthy and diseased periodontal tissues. Periodontology 2000 2006;40:29–49.
45. Hammerle CH, Giannobile WV, Working Group 1 of the European Workshop on Periodontology. Biology of soft tissue wound healing and regeneration– consensus report of Group 1 of the 10th European Workshop on Periodontology. J Clin Periodontol 2014;41(Suppl 15):S1–5.
46. Sculean A, Gruber R, Bosshardt DD. Soft tissue wound healing around teeth and dental implants. J Clin Periodontol 2014;41(Suppl 15):S6–22.
47. Tavelli L, McGuire MK, Zucchelli G, et al. Extracellular matrix-based scaffolding technologies for periodontal and peri-implant soft tissue regeneration. J Periodontol 2020;91:17–25.
48. Mancini L, Romandini M, Fratini A, et al. Biomaterials for periodontal and peri-implant regeneration. Materials (Basel) 2021;14(12):3319.
49. Tavelli L, Ravida A, Barootchi S, et al. Recombinant human platelet-derived growth factor: a systematic review of clinical findings in oral regenerative procedures. JDR Clin Trans Res 2021;6:161–73.
50. Albuquerque-Souza E, Schulte F, Chen T, et al. Maresin-1 and resolvin e1 promote regenerative properties of periodontal ligament stem cells under inflammatory conditions. Front Immunol 2020;11:585530.
51. Novello S, Pellen-Mussi P, Jeanne S. Mesenchymal stem cell-derived small extracellular vesicles as cell-free therapy: perspectives in periodontal regeneration. J Periodontal Res 2021;56:433–42.
52. Dieterle MP, Husari A, Steinberg T, et al. From the matrix to the nucleus and back: mechanobiology in the light of health, pathologies, and regeneration of oral periodontal tissues. Biomolecules 2021;11(6):824.

Decontamination and Biomodification of Periodontally Affected Root Surface for Successful Regeneration

Is There Room for Improvement?

Jamil Awad Shibli, DDS, MSc, PhD*, Magda Feres, DDS, MSc, DMSc,
Luciene C. Figueiredo, DDS, MSc, PhD,
Nidia Castro dos Santos, DDS, MSc, PhD*,
Belen Retamal-Valdes, DDS, MSc, PhD

KEYWORDS

- Periodontal diseases • Guided tissue regeneration • Root conditioning
- Root surface decontamination • Root coverage • Gingival recession
- Infraosseous defects • Laser

KEY POINTS

- Root modifiers do not provide clinical benefits for decontamination and biomodification of periodontally affected root surfaces.
- The use of enamel matrix derivative might improve clinical outcomes after the surgical treatment of deep intrabony defects.
- Standardized clinical trials in large populations, assessing biological and patient-reported outcome measures are necessary, to evaluate candidate biomaterials for decontamination and biomodification of periodontally affected root surfaces.

INTRODUCTION

Periodontitis is a multifactorial inflammatory condition associated with an oral microbiome dysbiosis that results in clinical attachment loss.[1] Nonsurgical and surgical therapies have been used to treat periodontitis, focusing on stopping further attachment loss and reestablish the clinical health condition. Scaling and root planing (SRP) is applied to all periodontitis cases to disturb the bacterial biofilm and remove

Department of Periodontology and Oral Implantology, Dental Research Division, Guarulhos University, Praça Tereza Cristina 229, Centro, Guarulhos, São Paulo 07023-070, Brazil
* Corresponding authors.
E-mail addresses: jshibli@ung.br (J.A.S.); nidia.castro@ymail.com (N.C.S.)

Dent Clin N Am 66 (2022) 11–38
https://doi.org/10.1016/j.cden.2021.06.001
dental.theclinics.com

calculus and any contaminated cementum.[2,3] Debridement of root surfaces using hand instruments or ultrasonic scalers results in a variated range of damage to the root surface. The root surface may also be exposed after debridement, and this factor may jeopardize future periodontal regeneration procedures.

The periodontal wound healing regeneration starts with the blood clot that functions as a matrix for the migration of inflammatory cells such as neutrophils and monocytes. This cascade of cellular events involves migration, adhesion, proliferation, and differentiation of several cell populations.[4] Thus, the decontamination and biomodification of root surfaces in combination with mechanical debridement to benefit periodontal healing is still a matter of debate. In that sense, several studies[5–7] have used strategies to modify or conditionate the periodontally affected root surface to increase tissue regeneration and root coverage success rates. Chemical, mechanical, and physical strategies[8–10] have been evaluated for their potential to modulate the hypermineralized surface layer and to remove the endotoxins. In general, promising results have been demonstrated in in vitro studies, although clinical trials have shown contradictory results.

Therefore, this narrative review aimed to address whether different root decontamination and/or biomodification methods could improve the periodontal regeneration of infrabone defects and root coverage. A search strategy was conducted as presented in **Box 1**. The related literature of clinical studies is discussed, and the future role of these strategies in periodontal regeneration is explored.

ROOT SURFACE MODIFIER STRATEGIES TO TREAT PERIODONTALLY AFFECTED TEETH

SRP can decrease and disturb the organization of bacterial dental biofilm and the cytotoxic substances contained in the calculus and cementum on root surfaces of periodontally diseased teeth. However, these procedures inevitably leave a smear layer that, with the remaining contaminated cementum, may negatively influence the recruiting and adhesion of periodontal ligament cells and inhibit new attachment.[11]

Box 1
Search strategy to root surface decontamination for tissue regeneration used in the PubMed database

Field 1: root surface, root surface modification, root surface biomodification, decontamination.

Field 2: tissue regeneration, intrabony defects, intrabony defects, infrabony defects, infrabony defects, intraosseous defects, intraosseous defects, vertical defects, furcation, furcation defects, furcation lesions, root coverage, periodontal defect.

Inclusion criteria: Surgical periodontal therapy, human study with periodontal clinical evaluation; sample size - 10 defects and/or teeth per group; present a negative control group (without root conditioner/root decontamination); 6-month follow-up

Exclusion criteria: in vitro studies; animal studies; case reports; histologic human reports; microbiological and immunologic studies without periodontal evaluation.

Biochemical agents:
   Citric acid, EDTA, Tetracycline, aPDT.

Mechanical and Physical agents:
   Polishing, Air polishing, Washing with saline solution, SRP, and Laser.

Possible antimicrobial effects:
   Emdogain, PRP, PRF.

Earlier studies[11–15] performed in the 1980s and 1990s evaluated the smear layer removal etching the denude root dentin and some portions of cementum with tetra-cycline hydrochloride, citric and phosphoric acids as well texapon detergent ethylenediaminetetra-acetic acid (EDTA). These modifiers also exposed dentinal tubules and reduced the endotoxins into the cementum. However, acidic modifiers resulted in a necrotizing effect on the surrounding tissues compared with EDTA treatment with a neutral pH and calcium chelator.[16] This chelating agent also preserved the integrity of exposed collagen fibers, early cell colonization, and vitality of adjacent tissues. In addition to etching chemical substances, some elegant reviews[17,18] showed that treated root sur-face by physical methods as laser and antimicrobial photodynamic therapy (aPDT) demonstrated better attachment of the regenerated periodontal tissues. erbium-doped yttrium-aluminium-garnet (Er:YAG) and erbium, chromium-doped yttrium-scandium-gallium-garnet (Er,Cr:YSGG) were used to improve the capability to remove and to condi-tioned the contaminated root surface for periodontal tissue regeneration.

Several attempts have been made to enhance regeneration outcomes by combining/adding root modifiers and membranes and/or barriers, as presented else-where in this article.

ROOT SURFACE MODIFIER STRATEGIES TO IMPROVE CLINICAL OUTCOMES OF PERIODONTAL SURGERIES

The multifactorial etiology of periodontitis and the several local and systemic risk factors associated with this disease makes periodontal tissue regeneration is a challenging task. Anti-infective and regenerative procedures have been evaluated in several inves-tigations for their capacity to remove as much as possible the contaminated cement and endotoxins. The ultimate goal of these studies were to assess the potential of these pro-cedures to modulate the regeneration of the lost periodontal tissues (**Table 1**).

Citric acid was the main root conditioner in the early 1980s. In vitro studies showed that root surfaces treated with a topical application of citric acid in different concen-trations and durations were able to remove the smear layer, expose collagen fibers, and enhance cell adhesion. However, translational studies[19,20] did not confirm these results, failing to show any differences between treatments with or without citric acid. Clinical studies evaluated the topical application of citric acid on furcation defects dur-ing periodontal anti-infective[19] or regenerative[20] surgeries. The results showed that citric acid promoted a "slight" or "weak" clinical improvement. There were no statis-tically significant differences in clinical periodontal parameters among the treatments using or not this substance.

Citric acid was also combined with surgical periodontal therapy to treat intrabony defects. The studies compared the effect of citric acid with those obtained by the application of saline solution, on shallow and deep periodontal pockets. Smith and colleagues (1986)[21] and Moore and colleagues (1987)[22] treated severe periodontitis patients with different flap surgery approaches and concluded that the anti-infective treatment *per se* was effective irrespective of the use of citric acid. Kersten and col-leagues (1992)[23] evaluated the adjunctive effect of conditioning root surfaces with cit-ric acid and guided tissue regeneration. A total of 26 periodontal defects with interproximal residual probing depth (PD) of 6 mm or greater with an intrabony defect of 4 mm or greater were divided into 2 groups: expanded polytetrafluoroethylene membrane with (test) or without (control) citric acid. At 12 months after treatment, both groups showed similar clinical improvements (*P*>.05).

Etching contaminated root surface with tetracycline HCl was also a commonly used strategy used mostly in the 1990s. The claim for this treatment protocol was that the

Table 1
Characteristics of studies that evaluated periodontal surgery and root surface decontamination

Study (Year)/ Root Modifier	Study Design	Follow-up Period (mo)	No of Treated Tooth/ No. of Treated Participants	Methodology	Clinical Outcomes	Conclusion
Parodi & Esper[19] (1984)/citric acid	Case control	6	20 lower molars with furcation involvement divided in test (topically applied citric acid) and control (saline solution)/there was no mention for number of patients	After 30 d of non-surgical periodontal therapy, the molars were divided in test (citric acid) and control (saline solution) and surgical periodontal procedures were performed in both groups. Clinical parameters were taken at pre-baseline, baseline, 3, and 6-mo postoperatively. Reentry was performed at 6 mo to measure bone level.	At 6-mo period: Proximal area: Test control ΔCAL 1.20 $\pm$ 0.65 1.06 $\pm$ 0.65 Furcation area: ΔCAL 1.00 $\pm$ 0.45 1.44 $\pm$ 0.72 Non-significant difference between groups (P>.05). Proximal area: Test control ΔBL 1.00 $\pm$ 0.37 0.58 $\pm$ 0.63 Furcation area: ΔBL 1.00 $\pm$ 0.45 0.92 $\pm$ 0.61 Nonsignificant difference between groups (P>.05).	The use of citric acid presented a "weak" beneficial effect in the furcation-involved human molars.

| Smith et al,[21] 1986/citric acid | Randomized | 6 | 120 teeth/10 participants with severe periodontitis | Teeth were divided in test (citric acid) and control (saline solution). Each are must present ≥2 teeth from second molar to cuspid, with PD ranged from 1 to 13 mm. Surgical access using modified Widman flap to scaling and root planning. The participants were included in a maintenance control during 2-, 4-, and 6-wk postsurgical for professional control. | At 6 mo period: All surfaces Shallow pockets (1 to 3 mm) Demonstrate clinical attachment loss for both groups (P>.05). Test control ΔCAL -0.31 ± 0.37– 0.25 ± 0.53 Pockets > 4 mm Demonstrate clinical attachment gain for both groups (P>.05). Test control ΔCAL 0.93 ± 0.80 0.30 ± 0.64 Interproximal surfaces Shallow pockets (1– 3 mm) Demonstrate clinical attachment loss for both groups (P>.05). Test control ΔCAL -0.39 ± 0.54– 0.34 ± 0.73 Pockets >4 mm Demonstrate clinical attachment gain for both groups (P>.05). | The citric acid did not clinical evidence of improve or accelerate periodontal healing during modified Widman flap surgery. CAL demonstrated similar patters for the groups in both shallow and moderate/deeper pockets. |

(continued on next page)

Table 1
(continued)

Study (Year)/ Root Modifier	Study Design	Follow-up Period (mo)	No of Treated Tooth/ No. of Treated Participants	Methodology	Clinical Outcomes	Conclusion
					Test control ΔCAL 0.12 ± 0.77 0.20 ± 0.73 Furcation defects: both groups showed decrease in the PD, although there was no difference statistical significance between groups ($P>.05$).	
Moore et al,[22] 1987/citric acid	Double-blind, controlled clinical trial on a split-mouth design	9	There was no mention for number of teeth/12	12 participants received initial periodontal therapy including oral hygiene instruction, SRP, and after a minimum period of 8 wk. Follow the initial therapy, 10 participants were included: present at least a pair of sites (except molars) with PD > 5 mm receive periodontal surgery	At baseline Test. Control CAL 7.58 + 1.10 7.38 ± 1.15 At 3 mo Test Control CAL 1.00 ± 1.15 1.17 ± 1.07 At 9 mo Test Control CAL 1.05 ± 1.60 0.90 ± 0.34 The test group presented gain of CAL in both 3	This study showed that 75% and 60% of experimental sites gain attachment at 3 and 9 mo irrespective of the treatment group. In addition, there was no statistical difference in all clinical parameters in the group of root surface etching with or

Study/year/agent	Study type	Number/defects	Methods	Results	Conclusions
			with adjunctive procedures: Test (citric acid with pH = 0.6) and control (saline solution). The participants also received penicillin and chlorhexidine 0.2%.	and 9m; control group did not (P<.05) PD and recession were improved at 3 and 9 mo for both groups, without difference between them (P>.05).	without citric acid during flap surgery.
Kersten et al,[23] 1992/citric acid	Randomized clinical study	12	26 intrabony defects/23	Defects with proximal residual PD ≥ 6 mm and intrabony defects ≥4 mm; the defects were surgically treated with test - citric acid and ePTFE and control – ePTFE without acid etching	At 12 mo period both groups showed similar clinical improvements (P>.05). Control test ΔCAL 1.0 ± 1.1 0.7 ± 1.5 ΔPD 1.8 ± 1.2 1.8 ± 1.2	The ePTFE barrier was effective to treat the defects irrespective the use of citric acid.
Fuentes et al,[20] 1993/citric acid	Clinical study	12	27 furcation defects/16	Patients with ≥1 mandibular molar with buccal class II furcation defect with horizontal PD >3 mm; Surgical treatment included coronal flap positioning with citric acid (test) or without (control).	At 12 mo period both groups showed similar clinical improvements (P>.05). Control test ΔCAL 0.4 ± 1.0 0.7 ± 1.1 Vertical and horizontal reentry bone fill ranged between 0.4 ± 1.0 and 1.8 ± 0.4 mm	Although a slight clinical improvement was associated with citric acid group without statistical significance, etching root surfaces may be not be "necessary part" of this procedure.

(continued on next page)

Table 1
(continued)

Study (Year)/ Root Modifier	Study Design	Follow-up Period (mo)	No of Treated Tooth/ No. of Treated Participants	Methodology	Clinical Outcomes	Conclusion
Machtei et al,[24] 1993/tetracycline HCl	RCT	12	36 furcation defects/18	Class II furcation involvement of the mandibular first or second molars were surgically treated with ePTFE; defects were treated with tetracycline HCl (test) or saline solution (control).	All clinical parameters were improved after treatment in both groups (*P*>.05). Tetracycline saline ΔPD 3.12 ± 1.5 3.16 ± 1.6 Microbiological differences were not detected between groups; however, *Actinobacillus actinomycetemcomitans* was detected in 5 sites during the monitoring phase and was associated with less favorable clinical results.	Anti-infective therapy and monitoring for *A actinomycetemcomitans* and/or other periodontal pathogens might be useful in guided tissue regeneration; tetracycline HCl did not improved the periodontal parameters.
Mayfield et al,[27] 1998/EDTA	CCS	6	36 interproximal intraosseous defects/36	3 mo after of hygienic treatment phase: Test group: access flap procedure + root conditioning with EDTA gel for 3 min followed by copious irrigation with sterile saline. Control group: access flap procedure	Test (mean ± SD) ΔPPD: 2.9 ± 1.3 ΔPAL: 1.8 ± 1.5 ΔGL: 1.1 ± 0.8 ΔPBL: 1.0 ± 1.3 % of defect remaining: 65% ± 30% Control (mean ± SD) ΔPPD: 2.6 ± 1.5 ΔPAL: 1.0 ± 1.7 ΔGL: 1.8 ± 0.7 ΔPBL: 0.4 ± 1.2 % of defect remaining: 73% ± 32%	EDTA gel did not provide additional benefits to flap surgery in the treatment of periodontal intraosseous defects.

| Issa et al,[28] 2019/ PBM-SMV-EDTA | RCT | 9 | 40 periodontal defects/40 | 4 wk after of hygienic treatment phase: Group 1: OFD, 1.2% SMV gel followed by defect coverage with OM. Group 2: OFD, 1.2% SMV gel, and defect coverage with PBM. Group 3: OFD, 24% EDTA root surface etching, 1.2% SMV gel, and coverage of the defect with OM. Group 4: OFD, 24% EDTA root surface etching, 1.2% SMV gel, and defect coverage with PBM. | Group 1
PPD BL: 6.2 ± 0.4
PPD 9M: 2.8 ± 0.4
CAL BL: 6.3 ± 0.6
CAL 9M: 3.0 ± 0.4
DBL BL: 6.5 ± 1.7
DBL 9M: 4.7 ± 1.0
CBL BL: 3.1 ± 1.1
CBL 9M: 3.2 ± 1.0
BD BL: 77.0 ± 9.0
BD 9M: 92.3 ± 6.8
Group 2
PPD BL: 6.2 ± 0.4
PPD 9M: 2.5 ± 0.5
CAL BL: 6.5 ± 0.7
CAL 9M: 3.2 ± 0.7
DBL BL: 6.3 ± 1.0
DBL 9M: 2.9 ± 1.0
CBL BL: 2.6 ± 0.6
CBL 9M: 2.2 ± 0.6
BD BL: 76.6 ± 12.7
BD 9M: 96.0 ± 11.9
Group 3
PPD BL: 6.3 ± 0.6
PPD 9M: 1.6 ± 0.5
CAL BL: 6.3 ± 0.6
CAL 9M: 1.8 ± 0.4
DBL BL: 6.1 ± 0.9
DBL 9M: 3.6 ± 0.7
CBL BL: 2.5 ± 0.5
CBL 9M: 1.8 ± 0.6
BD BL: 78.8 ± 12.4
BD 9M: 96.8 ± 11.1 | PBM-SMV-EDTA combination therapy seemed to be a promising regimen in treating periodontal defects. SMV availability seemed to be enhanced after the use of EDTA root surface etching. |

(continued on next page)

Table 1
(continued)

Study (Year)/ Root Modifier	Study Design	Follow-up Period (mo)	No of Treated Tooth/ No. of Treated Participants	Methodology	Clinical Outcomes	Conclusion
					Group 4	
					PPD BL: 6.3 ± 0.6	
					PPD 9M: 1.6 ± 0.7	
					CAL BL: 6.4 ± 0.7	
					CAL 9M: 2.0 ± 0.6	
					DBL BL: 6.5 ± 0.9	
					DBL 9M: 2.2 ± 0.8	
					CBL BL: 3.0 ± 0.7	
					CBL 9M: 2.2 ± 0.6	
					BD BL: 81.6 ± 9.3	
					BD 9M: 101.1 ± 6.9	
Cortellini et al,[31] 2007/EMD	COS	12	13 intrabony defects/13	3 mo after of hygienic treatment phase: MIST + EMD	PPD BL: 7.7 ± 1.8 PPD 12M: 2.9 ± 0.8 REC BL: 1.0 ± 1.5 REC 12M: 0.9 ± 2.1 CAL BL: 8.7 ± 2.7 CAL 12M: 3.8 ± 2.2	MIST associated with EMD is effective in the treatment of isolated deep intrabony defects.
Aslan et al,[32] 2017/EMD	COS	12	12 deep intrabony defects/12	3 mo after of hygienic treatment phase: EPP technique + 24% EDTA gel for 2 min + EMD	PPD BL: 9.7 ± 3.0 PPD 12M: 2.7 ± 0.7 REC BL: 2.5 ± 1.3 REC 12M: 2.66 ± 1.5 CAL BL: 12.2 ± 3.6 CAL 12M: 5.4 ± 2.0	EPP technique and 24% EDTA and EMD resulted in enhanced clinical outcomes in deep intrabony defects without any soft tissue complication

| Cosgarea et al,[33] 2021/air polishing | RCT | 12 | A total of 27 teeth (n = 14 test and n = 13 control)/30 patients with periodontitis stages III and IV were included at baseline; 27 participants were evaluated at 12 mo: n = 14 test and n = 13 control groups Smokers were also included | Single-center, examiner-masked, 2-arm parallel design RCT pilot study to compare clinical outcomes and side effects of root surface decontamination during periodontal surgery Test group: erythritol powder and air-polishing device (mid water and power settings for 10 s; Air-Flow Master with Perio-Flow System, EMS, Nyon, Switzerland) Control group: flap debridement using conventional hand and ultrasonic instruments | Primary outcome variable was CAL gain, with the patient as unit. Secondary endpoints were mean changes in FMPS, bleeding on probing, GBI, PD, decrease in the PD, CAL-, BS- (ΔBS) and BL-gain (ΔRBL) at 12 mo. All parameters decrease at 6 and 12 mo after therapy for both groups (P>.05); Reductions after 12 mo Test control ΔPD 3.00 ± 0.96 3.38 ± 1.12 ΔCAL 2.50 ± 1.60 2.85 ± 1.21 Nonsignificant difference between groups (P>.05). | Air polishing with an erythritol powder during periodontal surgery may represent a valuable minimally invasive adjunct following calculus removal by means of hand and ultrasonic instruments or a valuable alternative to these, for root surfaces without calculus. |

(continued on next page)

Table 1
(continued)

Study (Year)/ Root Modifier	Study Design	Follow-up Period (mo)	No of Treated Tooth/ No. of Treated Participants	Methodology	Clinical Outcomes	Conclusion
Clem et al,[36] 2020/Er, Cr:YSGG	RCT	6	79 intrabony defects/53	Multicenter, blinded study; patients with generalized periodontitis stage III, grade B; ≥1, but up to 2, nonadjacent teeth PD ≥6 mm and an intrabony defect with vertical dimension ≥3 mm; the defects were treated according to the group - Er,Cr:YSGG or MIST; PROs for pain, bleeding, swelling, ice pack use, anxiety, and satisfaction were also recorded.	After 6 mo period, both treatments presented similar results (P>.05) Er,Cr:YSGG MIST ΔCAL 1.26 ± 1.20 1.22 ± 1.32 ΔPPD 1.71 ± 1.18 1.63 ± 1.22 ΔGL - 0.41 ± 0.65– 0.35 ± 0.66 Er,Cr:YSGG group presented less bruising, facial swelling, and use of ice pack	Both treatments presented similar clinical outcomes, however superior effect in PROs for the surgical treatment of intrabony defects.

Karthikeyan et al,[37] 2019/diode	RCT	6	40 quadrants/20 patients	Patients with generalized chronic periodontitis PD ≥ 5 mm; 30% of sites with 3 ≤ CAL ≤ 5 mm; 6 teeth per quadrant Treatment groups: Kirkland flap surgery and DL-assisted open flap debridement (test) and Kirkland flap surgery (control). Microbiological test for the pathogens from red complex were also evaluated.	Test group presented better outcomes when compared with control group at 6 mo ($P<.001$) Test control ΔCAL 4.68 ± 1.02 3.14 ± 0.86 ΔPPD 4.72 ± 0.93 3.11 ± 0.90 The microbial reduction was statistically higher in the test group ($P<.05$).	Diode laser associated with Kirkland flap showed better clinical improvements than control group.
Martins et al,[40] 2017/aPDT	RCT	5	20 patients (unit of analysis)	Patients with interproximal attachment loss involving ≥2 contralateral teeth with PD ≥5 mm, CAL ≥5 mm and bleeding on probing. The defects were treated with flap debridement and aPDT (test) and flap debridement (control). Microbiological evaluation using DNA–DNA checkerboard hybridization.	aPDT improved statistically the periodontal parameters after 5 mo ($P<.001$) Test Control CAL 3.70 ± 0.80 4.18 ± 0.66 PPD 3.40 ± 0.50 2.70 ± 0.30 Beneficial microbial changes were positively associated with flap debridement + aPDT	Flap debridement associated with a single episode of aPDT presented beneficial results for the periodontal treatment.

(continued on next page)

Table 1
(continued)

Study (Year)/ Root Modifier	Study Design	Follow-up Period (mo)	No of Treated Tooth/ No. of Treated Participants	Methodology	Clinical Outcomes	Conclusion
Dilsiz et al,[48] 2010/Nd: YAG + EMD	RCT/split mouth design	12	41 intrabony defects/21	Intrabony defects without furcation involvement in each of 2 contralateral quadrants; PD ≥ 6 mm and depth of the defect component >3 mm. Defects were divided in test (Nd:YAG and EMD) and control (EMD) groups	At 12 mo follow-up, there was no statistical difference for periodontal parameters between groups (P>.05). Test control CAL 2.6 ± 1.2 3.0 ± 1.1 PPD 4.0 ± 0.8 4.4 ± 0.9	Nd:YAG laser root conditioning did not improve the outcome of EMD
Sculean et al,[35] 2004/Er:YAG	RCT	6	23 defects (Test n = 12; Control n = 11)/23	Intrabony defect with a PD ≥ 6 mm at interproximal sites; intrabony component of ≥3 mm as detected on radiographs. Defects were divided in Test (Er:YAG) and Control (flap debridement)	Test group Baseline 6 mo PD 7.8 ± 1.3 4.1 ± 1.3 (P<.05) CAL 9.8 ± 2.9 7.2 ± 2.5 (P<.05) Control group Baseline 6 mo PD 7.8 ± 0.8 4.6 ± 1.6 (P<.05) CAL 9.1 ± 1.2 7.7 ± 1.6 (P<.05) Test and control groups present no statistical differences at 6 mo period.	Er:YAG laser did not improve the clinical outcomes.

| Schwarz et al,[39] 2003/Er:YAG and EMD | RCT | 6 | 42 intrabony defects/22 | Intrabony defect with a PD ≥ 6 mm at interproximal sites; intrabony component of ≥3 mm as detected on radiographs. Defects were treated with EMD associated (test) or not (control) with Er:YAG | The association of EMD and Er:YAG laser did not improve the clinical outcomes (P>.05). Test group Baseline 6 mo PD 8.1 ± 0.8 4.0 ± 0.5 (P<.001) CAL 10.4 ± 1.1 7.1 ± 1.2 (P<.001) Control group Baseline 6 mo PD 8.6 ± 1.2 4.6 ± 0.8 (P<.001) CAL 10.7 ± 1.3 7.5 ± 1.4 (P<.001) | Both therapies led to short-term improvements of clinical parameters, however, Er:YAG laser did not add additional benefit to the treatment. |

Abbreviations: ΔGL, gingival level change; ΔPBL, probing bone level change; ΔPPD, probing pocket depth change; BD, bone density; BL, baseline; CAL, clinical attachment level; CBL, crestal bone level; CC, case-control studies; COS, cohort studies; CS, case series; DBL, defect base level; EMD, enamel matrix derivative; EPP, entire papilla preservation; ePTFE, expanded polytetrafluoroethylene; GIB, gingival bleeding index; MIST, minimally invasive surgical technique; OFD, open flap debridement; OM, occlusive membranes; PAL, probing attachment level change; PBM, perforated barrier membrane; PPD, probing pocket depth; RCT, randomized clinical trials; REC, recession of the gingival margin; SD, standard deviation; SMV, simvastatin.

bacteriostatic effect of tetracycline against periodontal pathogens would potentiate the effects of mechanical therapy. Machtei and colleagues (1993)[24] evaluated the clinical and microbiological effects of topic tetracycline to treat class II furcation involvement on mandibular molars. All furcation defects were treated with expanded polytetrafluoroethylene and tetracycline HCl (test) or saline solution (control). All clinical parameters were improved after treatment in both groups, with mean PD decrease ranging between 3.12 ± 1.5 mm and 3.16 ± 1.6 mm for tetracycline and saline solution, respectively (P>.05). The authors also pointed out that microbiological differences were not detected between groups.

Later studies[11,25,26] focused on different substances with neutral or basic pH to avoid undesired effects of acidic conditioners, mainly on the necrosis of the periodontal tissues. One of the substances tested was EDTA, an organic compound that acts as a chemical chelator for Ca^{+2} ions present in the root surfaces. Several in vitro and animal studies[11,25,26] indicated that root surfaces conditioned with EDTA gel (24%, pH 7) depicted a smear-free root surface. The exposed collagen fibrins provided a biocompatible surface for periodontal tissue healing compared with a mineralized root surface covered with the smear layer. These preliminary findings encouraged other researchers to evaluate the periodontal clinical outcomes after periodontal surgeries. Unfortunately, overall, the clinical studies were not able to confirm the encouraging in vitro and animal studies. Mayfield and colleagues (1998)[27] conducted a case control study to compare the clinical effect of access flap procedure and root conditioning using EDTA to treat intraosseous periodontal defects in periodontitis patients. Three months after the hygienic treatment phase, 1 interproximal intraosseous defect with a PD ≥ 5 mm and bleeding on probing per volunteer was assigned to the surgical phase. In the test group (n = 18), after access flap procedure and careful debridement and root planing, the EDTA gel preparation was applied to the root surface for 3 minutes and followed by copious irrigation with sterile saline solution. The control group (n = 18) was treated using an access flap alone. Six months after surgery, it was concluded that EDTA gel did not provide additional benefits to flap surgery to treat intraosseous defects.

Recently, Issa and colleagues (2020)[28] conducted a clinical study to evaluate the clinical and radiographic outcomes following the use of a novel perforated barrier membrane (PBM) and simvastatin (SMV) gel compared with SMV gel and traditional occlusive membranes in both EDTA-treated and nontreated patients. All volunteers were recalled 4 weeks after hygienic periodontal therapy, and a clinical reevaluation was performed to confirm the need for guided tissue reconstructive surgery using membranes in selected teeth. To be assigned to surgery a tooth had to have 1 interproximal site with a PD ≥ 5 mm, clinical attachment level (CAL) of at least 4 mm and interproximal intrabony defects of at least 3 mm. The participants were randomly assigned to 4 groups (10 patients each) receiving the following treatments: (i) group 1: open flap debridement, 1.2% SMV gel followed by defect coverage with an occlusive membrane; (ii) group 2: open flap debridement and 1.2% SMV gel followed by defect coverage with PBM; (ii) group 3: open flap debridement, 24% EDTA root surface etching, 1.2% SMV gel, and coverage of the defect with an occlusive membrane; and (iv) group 4: open flap debridement, 24% EDTA root surface etching, 1.2% SMV gel, and defect coverage with PBM. Clinical and radiographic parameters were measured 1 week before and 6 months after the surgical procedures. The authors concluded that using PBM–SMV–EDTA combination therapy seemed to be a promising regimen in treating periodontal defects and SMV availability seemed to be enhanced after the use of EDTA root surface etching.

The lack of clinical evidence to support the use of root decontamination modifiers as adjunctive to the periodontal treatment raises concern about the potential of recruitment of periodontal cells during wound healing. Guided tissue regeneration improved periodontal tissue regeneration procedures with a gain of periodontal attachment based on the selective exclusion of epithelial cells from colonizing the wound and space-maintaining for the blood clot regenerate lost periodontal tissues. Emdogain is an enamel matrix derivative (EMD) composed of several proteins, mostly amelogenins. These proteins are thought to induce the formation of the periodontal attachment during tooth formation, and its application on affected periodontally root surface may have a similar property during periodontal wound healing.[29] A preclinical study[30] evaluated the effect of protein fractions of the matrix on periodontal regeneration in a buccal dehiscence model in monkeys, showing new periodontal attachment formation in contrast with the control side that received no treatment.

Prospective cohort human clinical studies were conducted in the treatment of intrabony defects using EMD. Cortellini and colleagues (2007)[31] treated 13 patients with the minimally invasive surgical technique associated with the application of EMD in the treatment of isolated deep intrabony defects. Participants received periodontal treatment and, at 3 months after the hygienic treatment phase, they received the regenerative surgery with minimally invasive surgical technique + EMD. The case cohort demonstrated the potential efficacy of minimally invasive surgical technique associated with EMD in the treatment of isolated deep intrabony defects.[31]

Aslan and colleagues (2017)[32] conducted a prospective cohort study to evaluate the clinical effects of entire papilla preservation technique plus 24% EDTA gel and EMD to treat isolated deep intrabony defects in 12 participants. Three months after completion of a hygienic phase, 1 or more deep intrabony defect per patient received regenerative periodontal treatment using the study protocol. All volunteers received a clinical periodontal assessment at 3 months after the hygienic periodontal phase and 12 months after the regenerative periodontal surgery. The authors concluded that the entire papilla preservation technique and 24% EDTA plus EMD resulted in enhanced clinical outcomes in deep intrabony defects without any soft tissue complication.

Air polishing has also been studied as a possible adjunctive treatment to surgical periodontal therapy. Cosgarea and colleagues (2021)[33] conducted a parallel single-center pilot randomized clinical trial (RCT) that evaluated the use of erythritol powder and air-polishing devices in open flap periodontal surgery. A total of 27 participants with stages III and IV periodontitis presenting 1 experimental single-rooted tooth with a PD $\geq$ 6 mm and horizontal bone loss with a maximum of a 2-mm intrabony component as detected radiographically were included. Surgical treatment of the patients were divided into test (air-polishing) and control (hand and ultrasonic scalers) group and, showed no difference for the primary and secondary outcomes after 6 and 12 months of follow-up.

Many researchers have reported the use of laser as adjunctive to periodontal therapy[17,18]. High-power lasers as CO_2, Er:YAG, neodymium-doped yttrium-aluminum-garnet (Nd:YAG), and Er,Cr:YSGG are expensive tools that have been tested for a possible positive effect as adjuncts in periodontal therapy. A narrative review[34] also suggested that Er:YAG laser and some low-level lasers provided a secondary effect defined as photobiomodulation that improves the host-response after surgical procedures. In addition, aPDT has been used in periodontal therapy to improve the subgingival microbial composition, with different degrees of success. Photosensitizers are associated with the low-level laser to generate a free radical called oxygen singlet that can act specifically in some periodontal pathogens.[18] Several well-conducted clinical studies evaluated the adjunctive effect of laser with periodontal surgery procedures in the last decades. Er:YAG,[35] Er,Cr:YSGG[36] and diode[37] were associated with anti-infective surgical periodontal therapy to treat intrabony defects. Gain of attachment level and decrease of PD were demonstrated in all studies; however, the studies failed to present the results' superiority using lasers. Other studies[38,39] associated EMD after laser irradiation of the root surfaces, but this procedure did not improve attachment level gain or decreases in the PD.

Martins and colleagues (2017)[40] carried out a RCT comparing the use of a single application of aPDT in periodontal diseases' surgical treatment. A total of 20 patients with interproximal attachment loss involving 2 or more contralateral teeth with PD $\geq$ 5 mm, CAL $\geq$ 5 mm and bleeding on probing were divided into 2 groups: (i) test group: aPDT and surgical debridement, and (ii) control group: surgical debridement. Periodontal clinical parameters and microbiological samples were taken after 5 months postsurgically. The aPDT improved the periodontal parameters ($P<.001$) statistically and showed a beneficial microbial effect in the subgingival environment, at least after 5 months of follow-up.

ROOT SURFACE MODIFIER STRATEGIES TO ENHANCE ROOT COVERAGE PROCEDURES

Different root surface decontamination and modifier strategies have been investigated regarding their efficacy to improve the clinical outcomes of root coverage procedures (**Table 2**). Initially, tetracycline was suggested as a root surface modifier, combined with fibrin-fibronectin for guided tissue regeneration in a case series.[41] The authors reported that this root coverage procedure provided a mean attachment level gain of 4.5 $\pm$ 1.40 mm, a mean decrease in the PD of -0.90 ± 0.80 mm, and a mean root coverage was 77.4%. Because this study did not include a control group, the effectiveness of adjunctive tetracycline was not demonstrated when compared with surgical procedures alone.

In 2000, the use of citric acid and EDTA as adjuncts to root coverage procedures were investigated in 3 RCTs.[42–44] Caffesse and colleagues (2000)[42] investigated the use of citric acid as a root modifier for a subepithelial connective tissue graft (SCTG) compared with SCTG alone. No significant changes in PD were observed (-0.16 ± 0.06 mm vs -0.13 ± 0.81 mm). The authors concluded that citric acid did not affect the clinical outcomes of SCTG.[42]

Kassab and colleagues (2006)[43] hypothesized that EDTA as a root modifier could enhance root coverage after SCTG. The experimental sites received EDTA, and the control group received distilled water. The mean CAL was 1.90 $\pm$ 0.70 mm for the EDTA group and 1.60 $\pm$ 0.50 mm for the control group at 6 months. The mean decrease in the PD was the same for the EDTA and the control group at 6 months: 1.60 $\pm$ 0.50 mm. Thus, this study failed to show a benefit from EDTA use, over the benefits attained with SCTG only.

Bittencourt and colleagues (2007)[44] used EDTA gel as a root modifier before a semilunar coronally positioned flap (SCPF) procedure and compared with a control group without EDTA. At 6 months, the attachment level gain (1.25 $\pm$ 0.69 mm for EDTA + SCPF vs 1.60 $\pm$ 0.56 mm for SCPF) and decrease in PD (0.00 $\pm$ 0.45 mm for EDTA + SCPF vs -0.03 ± 0.29 mm for SCPF) did not present statistically significant differences for intergroup comparisons. Additionally, when recession height and width changes were compared between groups, statistically significant differences favoring the control group were observed. Therefore, the authors concluded that EDTA gel as a root surface modifier negatively affected the outcome of root coverage after SCPF.[44]

Table 2

Characteristics of studies that evaluated coverage procedures and root surface decontamination

Study (Year)/ Root Modifier	Study Design	Follow-up Period (mo)	No. of Treated Tooth/No. of Treated Participants	Methodology	Clinical Outcomes	Conclusion
Bittencourt et al,[44] 2007/EDTA	Split-mouth RCT	6	30/15	Test Semilunar coronally repositioned flap + 24% EDTA Control Semilunar coronally repositioned flap	Test CAL BL: 3.40 ± 0.61 mm CAL 6 mo: 2.15 ± 0.82 mm Overall change: 1.25 ± 0.69 mm PD BL: 1.53 ± 0.48 mm PD 6 mo: 1.53 ± 0.52 mm Overall change: 0.00 ± 0.45 mm Control CAL BL: 3.39 ± 0.77 mm CAL 6 mo: 1.79 ± 0.80 mm Overall change: 1.60 ± 0.56 mm PD BL: 1.60 ± 0.51 mm PD 6 mo: 1.63 ± 0.61 mm Overall change: −0.03 ± 0.29 mm	The use of EDTA negatively affected the outcome of root coverage with the semilunar coronally repositioned flap.
Caffesse et al,[42] 2000/Citric acid	RCT	6	36/36	Test Citric acid + SCTG Control SCTG	Test PD BL: 1.68 ± 0.48 mm PD 6 mo: 1.53 ± 0.61 mm Overall change: −0.16 ± 0.06 mm Control PD BL: 1.63 ± 0.62 mm PD 6 mo: 1.50 ± 0.73 mm Overall change: −0.13 ± 0.81 mm	Citric acid did not provide additional benefits to SCTG.

(continued on next page)

Table 2 (*continued*)

Study (Year)/Root Modifier	Study Design	Follow-up Period (mo)	No. of Treated Tooth/No. of Treated Participants	Methodology	Clinical Outcomes	Conclusion
Damante et al,[51] 2019/Citric acid, tetracyclines, aPDT	RCT	12	60/17 (n = 20/group)	Test 1 CA/tetracycline gel (CAT) + SRP Test2 aPDT + SRP Control SRP	Test 1 CAL BL: 3.23 ± 1.38 mm CAL 12M: 0.55 ± 1.68 mm PD BL: 1.30 ± 0.44 mm PD 12M: 1.45 ± 0.60 mm Test 2 CAL BL: 4.03 ± 1.30 mm CAL 12M: 0.80 ± 2.11 mm PD BL: 1.55 ± 0.63 mm PD 12M: 1.83 ± 0.85 mm Control CAL BL: 4.30 ± 1.03 mm CAL 12M: 2.50 ± 1.99 mm PD BL: 1.60 ± 0.68 mm PD 12M: 1.95 ± 0.94 mm	Root conditioning, with CAT or aPDT, promotes better long-term clinical outcomes and root coverage after SCTG procedures.
Dilsiz et al,[49] 2010/Laser	Split-mouth RCT	6	34/17	Test SCTG + Nd:YAG laser Control SCTG	Test CAL BL: 4.67 ± 1.33 mm CAL 6 mo: 3.75 ± 1.16 mm PD BL: 1.38 ± 0.51 mm PD 6 mo: 1.50 ± 0.50 mm Control CAL BL: 4.88 ± 1.12 mm CAL 6 mo: 2.33 ± 1.25 mm PD BL: 1.46 ± 0.63 mm PD 6 mo: 1.50 ± 0.50 mm	The use of Nd:YAG laser negatively affected the outcome of root coverage with the SCTG.

Study/Year/Topic	Study design	Follow-up (mo)	n	Intervention	Results	Conclusion
Dilsiz et al,[49] 2010/Laser	Split-mouth RCT	6	24/12	Test: SCTG + Er:YAG laser; Control: SCTG	Test — CAL BL: 4.54 ± 0.90 mm; CAL 6 mo: 2.04 ± 0.59 mm; PD BL: 1.46 ± 0.43 mm; PD 6 mo: 1.46 ± 0.66 mm. Control — CAL BL: 4.67 ± 0.94 mm; CAL 6 mo: 2.08 ± 0.49 mm; PD BL: 1.58 ± 0.49 mm; PD 6 mo: 1.63 ± 0.68 mm	Er:YAG laser did not provide additional benefits to SCTG.
Kassab et al,[43] 2000/EDTA	Split-mouth RCT	6	20/10	Test: 24% EDTA + CTG; Control: Distilled water + CTG	Test — CAL BL: 6.00 ± 0.70 mm; CAL 6 mo: 1.90 ± 0.70 mm; PD BL: 1.70 ± 0.50 mm; PD 6 mo: 1.60 ± 0.50 mm. Control — CAL BL: 5.60 ± 0.50 mm; CAL 6 mo: 1.60 ± 0.50 mm; PD BL: 1.60 ± 0.50 mm; PD 6 mo: 1.60 ± 0.50 mm	EDTA did not provide additional benefits.
Pini Prato et al,[47] 2011/Air Polishing	Follow-up of a split-mouth RCT	12	20/10	Test: Polishing + CAF; Control: SRP + CAF	Test — PD BL: 1.30 ± 0.50 mm; PD 12M: 0.70 ± 0.40 mm. Control — PD BL: 1.30 ± 0.50 mm; PD 12M: 1.00 ± 0.40 mm	The study did not report a comparative analysis for PD.

(continued on next page)

Table 2
(continued)

Study (Year)/ Root Modifier	Study Design	Follow-up Period (mo)	No. of Treated Tooth/No. of Treated Participants	Methodology	Clinical Outcomes	Conclusion
Poormoradi et al,[50] 2018/Laser	Split-mouth RCT	6	30/5	Test SCTG + Er, Cr:YSGG laser Control SCTG	Test CAL BL: 4.80 ± 1.20 mm CAL 6 mo: 1.33 ± 0.97 mm PD BL: 1.53 ± 0.64 mm PD 6 mo: 1.13 ± 0.35 mm Control CAL BL: 4.67 ± 1.11 mm CAL 6 mo: 1.80 ± 1.32 mm PD BL: 1.47 ± 0.64 mm PD 6 mo: 1.27 ± 0.45 mm	Er,Cr:YSGG laser did not provide CAL gain/ decrease in the PD to SCTG.
Roman et al,[58] 2013/Emdogain	RCT	12	42/42	Test SCTG + EMD Control SCTG	Test PD BL: 1.30 ± 0.56 mm PD 12M: 1.57 ± 0.51 mm Control PD BL: 1.59 ± 0.50 mm PD 6 mo: 1.55 ± 0.51 mm	EMD did not provide additional benefits to SCTG.
Trombelli et al,[41] 1994/Tetracycline	CS	6	15/15	Case Trapezium-shaped flap + Tetracycline HCl solution (100 mg/mL) + EePTFE membrane + fibrin-fibronectin sealing system	Case CAL BL: 6.50 ± 0.80 mm CAL 6 mo: 2.00 ± 1.40 mm Overall change: −4.5 ± 1.40 mm PD BL: 1.80 ± 0.60 mm PD 6 mo: 0.90 ± 0.50 mm Overall change: −0.90 ± 0.80 mm	The use of guided tissue regeneration plus tetracycline and fibrin-fibronectin provided improvement of mucogingival defects.

| Zucchelli et al,[45] 2009/Ultrasonic piezoelectric | Split-mouth RCT | 6 | 22/11 | Test
Ultrasonic piezoelectric instrumentation + CAF
Control
SRP + CAF | Test
CAL BL: 4.90 ± 0.54 mm
CAL 6 mo: 2.00 ± 0.63 mm
Overall change:
  2.90 ± 0.70 mm
PD BL: 1.09 ± 0.30 mm
PD 6 mo: 1.36 ± 0.50 mm
Overall change:
  0.27 ± 0.64 mm
Control
CAL BL: 4.72 ± 0.78 mm
CAL 6 mo: 1.36 ± 0.50 mm
Overall change:
  3.36 ± 0.92 mm
PD BL: 1.09 ± 0.09 mm
PD 6 mo: 1.18 ± 0.40 mm
Overall change:
  0.18 ± 0.40 mm | Ultrasonic piezoelectric instrumentation did not provide additional benefits to SCTG |

Abbreviations: BL, baseline; CS, case series; ePTFE, expanded polytetrafluoroethylene; RCT, randomized clinical trials; SCGT, subepithelial connective tissue graft.

Two split-mouth RCTs investigated different instrumentation approaches as root modifiers. Zucchelli and colleagues (2009)[45] used ultrasonic piezoelectric instrumentation preceding coronally advanced flap (CAF) compared with SRP and CAF. Six months after surgery, the mean attachment level gain was statistically significant in both groups (test, 2.90 ± 0.70 mm; control, 3.36 ± 0.92 mm), but without a difference between them (P>.05). Similarly, mean decrease in the PD did not differ between the test (0.27 ± 0.64 mm) and control (0.18 ± 0.40 mm) groups (P>.05). It was concluded that ultrasonic piezoelectric instrumentation did not show additional benefits for CAF compared with SRP.[45] Pini Prato and colleagues (2011)[46] presented the 14-year outcomes from a previously published split-mouth RCT with a follow-up of 3 months[47] that compared root surface polishing to root planning, used in combination with CAF. The overall mean changes in PD did not differ between test ad control groups over the course of the study. At 14 years of follow-up, mean decrease in the PD was 1.00 ± 0.60 mm and 1.00 ± 0.50 mm in the test and control groups, respectively. Although a comparative statistical analysis was not presented for this outcome, the raw numbers suggest no additional clinically relevant benefits for root polishing over those obtained with root planning.[46]

In the last decade, the use of lasers as root modifiers on root coverage procedures were investigated in 3 clinical trials.[48–50] Through split-mouth RCTs, Dilsiz and colleagues tested if the use of Nd:YAG laser[48] and Er:YAG laser[49] promoted additional benefits in combination with SCTG. When Nd:YAG laser was applied, mean CAL was 3.75 ± 1.16 mm for the test group and 2.33 ± 1.25 mm for the control group at 6 months after surgery. No statistically significant difference was detected when the study groups were compared. However, when the test and the control groups were compared for average root coverage (33% vs 77%, for test and control groups respectively) and complete root coverage (18% vs 65%, for test and control groups respectively), the results favored the control group. Therefore, it was concluded that Nd:YAG laser as a root modifier negatively affected the outcome of root coverage with the SCTG.[48] The use of Er:YAG laser as a root modifier was also tested in combination with SCTG. At 6 months, the mean CAL was 2.04 ± 0.59 mm for the test group and 2.08 ± 0.49 mm for the control group (P>.05). Average root coverage was 80% for the test group and 86% for the control group, and complete root coverage was 75% and 67%, respectively. The authors concluded that root surface conditioning with Er:YAG laser did not provide additional benefits for the SCTG technique.[49] Poormoradi and colleagues (2018)[50] evaluated the use of SCTG combined with Er,Cr:YSGG laser compared with SCTG alone in the clinical outcomes of root coverage procedures. After 6 months, no significant differences were observed in the assessed parameters when test and control groups were compared, including mean CAL (1.33 ± 0.97 mm vs 1.80 ± 1.32 mm, for test and control groups, respectively) and mean PD (1.13 ± 0.35 mm vs 1.27 ± 0.45 mm, for test and control groups, respectively).[50]

Damante and colleagues (2019)[51] investigated the use of root conditioning with aPDT compared with citric acid plus tetracycline gel and SRP. Seventeen patients were included in the study, and 60 recession defects were treated (n = 20/group). The patients were followed for 12 months. The aPDT group presented CA reduction and a higher percentage of complete root coverage when compared with SRP. The citric acid plus tetracycline gel group demonstrated a better decrease in CAL, PD, recession depth, and a higher rate of complete root coverage when compared with SRP. Therefore, it was concluded that root conditioning, with aPDT or citric acid plus tetracycline, promoted better clinical outcomes after SCTG procedures.[51]

FUTURE PERSPECTIVES

To date, studies evaluating the effectiveness of root surface decontamination and bio-modification methods in the treatment of periodontitis or root coverage procedures have focused on the biological outcomes of treatment (eg, clinical, microbiological, histologic) evaluated by the clinical investigator. However, there is a current trend an incentive to the assessment of the patients' perception of the success of different therapies in the health field.[52–55] To assess and to compare the level of knowledge, quality of life, and level of satisfaction of patients with dental treatment, researchers have used structured patient-reported outcome measures.[56,57] The results of research evaluating biological parameters and patient-reported outcome measures after dental procedures would be the most effective way to determine the use of new periodontal treatments in clinical practice, and can also guide the conduction of future investigations in the field.

SUMMARY

Research over the past decades does not support the use of root modifiers for decon-tamination and biomodification of periodontally affected root surfaces, neither for anti-infective surgical or regenerative treatments or for root coverage procedures. Several treatment approaches, from acidic modifiers to lasers, have been investigated and provided some limited additional clinically relevant benefits to periodontal procedures. Nevertheless, the studies suggested that EMD proteins might promote clinical bene-fits for the treatment of deep intrabony defects. Future studies testing EMD proteins, and assessing biological parameters together with patient-reported outcome mea-sures as outcomes of treatment are recommended.

CLINICS CARE POINTS

- Root modifiers failed to provide additional clinical benefits for decontamination and biomodification after periodontal surgeries.
- The use of enamel matrix derivative might improve clinical outcomes after the surgical treatment of deep intrabony defects.
- Evidence does not support the use of root modifiers to improve root coverage procedures.

DISCLOSURE

The authors have nothing to disclose.

REFERENCES

1. Papapanou PN, Sanz M, Buduneli N, et al. Periodontitis: consensus report of workgroup 2 of the 2017 World Workshop on the Classification of Periodontal and Peri-Implant Diseases and Conditions. J Clin Periodontol 2018;45(Suppl 20):S162–70.
2. Adriaens PA, De Boever JA, Loesche WJ. Bacterial invasion in root cementum and radicular dentin of periodontally diseased teeth in humans. A reservoir of pe-riodontopathic bacteria. J Periodontol 1988;59:222–30.
3. Carvalho LH, D'Avila GB, Leão A, et al. Scaling and root planing, systemic metro-nidazole and professional plaque removal in the treatment of chronic periodontitis in a Brazilian population. I. clinical results. J Clin Periodontol 2004;31:1070–6.

4. Grzesik WJ, Narayanan AS. Cementum and periodontal wound healing and regeneration. Crit Rev Oral Biol Med 2002;13:474–84.
5. Zandim DL, Leite FR, da Silva VC, et al. Wound healing of dehiscence defects following different root conditioning modalities: an experimental study in dogs. Clin Oral Investig 2013;17:1585–93.
6. Carvalho Batista LH, Cezar Sampaio JE, Pilatti GL, et al. Efficacy of EDTA-T gel for smear layer removal at root surfaces. Quintessence Int 2005;36:551–8.
7. Karam PS, Sant'Ana AC, de Rezende ML, et al. Root surface modifiers and sub-epithelial connective tissue graft for treatment of gingival recessions: a systematic review. J Periodont Res 2016;51:175–85.
8. Koop R, Merheb J, Quirynen M. Periodontal regeneration with enamel matrix derivative in reconstructive periodontal therapy: a systematic review. J Periodontol 2012;83:707–20.
9. Mariotti A. Efficacy of chemical root surface modifiers in the treatment of periodontal disease. A systematic review. Ann Periodontol 2003;8:205–26.
10. Behdin S, Monje A, Lin GH, et al. Effectiveness of laser application for periodontal surgical therapy: systematic review and meta-analysis. J Periodontol 2015;86:1352–63.
11. Blomlöf J, Lindskog S. Root surface texture and early cell and tissue colonization after different etching modalities. Eur J Oral Sci 1995;103:17–24.
12. Zappa UE. Factors determining the outcome of scaling and root planing. Probe 1992;26:152–9.
13. Polson AM, Ladenheim S, Hanes PJ. Cell and fiber attachment to demineralized dentin from periodontitis-affected root surfaces. J Periodontol 1986;57:235–46.
14. Polson AM, Hanes PJ. Cell and fiber attachment to demineralized dentin. A comparison between normal and periodontitis-affected root surfaces. J Clin Periodontol 1987;14:357–65.
15. Hanes P, Polson A, Frederick T. Citric acid treatment of periodontitis-affected cementum. A scanning electron microscopic study. J Clin Periodontol 1991;18:567–75.
16. Zaman KU, Sugaya T, Hongo O, et al. A study of attached and oriented human periodontal ligament cells to periodontally diseased cementum and dentin after demineralizing with neutral and low pH etching solution. J Periodontol 2000;71:1094–9.
17. Schwarz F, Aoki A, Sculean A, et al. The impact of laser application on periodontal and peri-implant wound healing. Periodontol 2000 2009;51:79–108.
18. Aoki A, Mizutani K, Schwarz F, et al. Periodontal and peri-implant wound healing following laser therapy. Periodontol 2000 2015;68:217–69.
19. Parodi RJ, Esper ME. Effect of topical application of citric acid in the treatment of furcation involvement in human lower molars. J Clin Periodontol 1984;11:644–51.
20. Fuentes P, Garrett S, Nilvéus R, et al. Treatment of periodontal furcation defects. Coronally positioned flap with or without citric acid root conditioning in class II defects. J Clin Periodontol 1993;20:425–30.
21. Smith BA, Mason WE, Morrison EC, et al. The effectiveness of citric acid as an adjunct to surgical re-attachment procedures in humans. J Clin Periodontol 1986;13:701–8.
22. Moore JA, Ashley FP, Waterman CA. The effect on healing of the application of citric acid during replaced flap surgery. J Clin Periodontol 1987;14:130–5.
23. Kersten BG, Chamberlain AD, Khorsandi S, et al. Healing of the intrabony periodontal lesion following root conditioning with citric acid and wound closure including an expanded PTFE membrane. J Periodontol 1992;63:876–82.

24. Machtei EE, Dunford RG, Norderyd OM, et al. Guided tissue regeneration and anti-infective therapy in the treatment of class II furcation defects. J Periodontol 1993;64:968–73.
25. Blomlöf J. Root cementum appearance in healthy monkeys and periodontitis-prone patients after different etching modalities. J Clin Periodontol 1996;23:12–8.
26. Blomlöf JP, Blomlöf LB, Lindskog SF. Smear removal and collagen exposure after non-surgical root planing followed by etching with an EDTA gel preparation. J Periodontol 1996;67:841–5.
27. Mayfield L, Söderholm G, Norderyd O, et al. Root conditioning using EDTA gel as an adjunct to surgical therapy for the treatment of intraosseous periodontal defects. J Clin Periodontol 1998;25:707–14.
28. Issa DR, Abdel-Ghaffar KA, Al-Shahat MA, et al. Guided tissue regeneration of intrabony defects with perforated barrier membranes, simvastatin, and EDTA root surface modification: a clinical and biochemical study. J Periodont Res 2020;55:85–95.
29. Hammarström L. Enamel matrix, cementum development and regeneration. J Clin Periodontol 1997;24:658–68.
30. Hammarström L, Heijl L, Gestrelius S. Periodontal regeneration in a buccal dehiscence model in monkeys after application of enamel matrix proteins. J Clin Periodontol 1997;24:669–77.
31. Cortellini P, Tonetti MS. A minimally invasive surgical technique with an enamel matrix derivative in the regenerative treatment of intra-bony defects: a novel approach to limit morbidity. J Clin Periodontol 2007;34:87–93.
32. Aslan S, Buduneli N, Cortellini P. Entire papilla preservation technique in the regenerative treatment of deep intrabony defects: 1-Year results. J Clin Periodontol 2017;44:926–32.
33. Cosgarea R, Jepsen S, Fimmers R, et al. Clinical outcomes following periodontal surgery and root surface decontamination by erythritol-based air polishing. A randomized, controlled, clinical pilot study. Clin Oral Investig 2021;25:627–35.
34. Arany PR. Craniofacial wound healing with photobiomodulation therapy: new insights and current challenges. J Dent Res 2016;95:977–84.
35. Sculean A, Schwarz F, Berakdar M, et al. Healing of intrabony defects following surgical treatment with or without an Er:YAG laser. J Clin Periodontol 2004;31:604–8.
36. Clem D, Heard R, McGuire M, et al. Comparison of Er,Cr:YSGG laser to minimally invasive surgical technique in the treatment of intrabony defects: six-month results of a multicenter, randomized, controlled study. J Periodontol 2021;92(4):496–506.
37. Karthikeyan J, Vijayalakshmi R, Mahendra J, et al. Diode Laser as an Adjunct to Kirkland Flap Surgery-A Randomized Split-Mouth Clinical and Microbiological Study. Photobiomodul Photomed Laser Surg 2019;37:99–109.
38. Dilsiz A, Canakci V, Aydin T. The combined use of Nd:YAG laser and enamel matrix proteins in the treatment of periodontal infrabony defects. J Periodontol 2010;81:1411–8.
39. Schwarz F, Sculean A, Georg T, et al. Clinical evaluation of the Er:YAG laser in combination with an enamel matrix protein derivative for the treatment of intrabony periodontal defects: a pilot study. J Clin Periodontol 2003;30:975–81.
40. Martins SHL, Novaes AB Jr, Taba M Jr, et al. Effect of surgical periodontal treatment associated to antimicrobial photodynamic therapy on chronic periodontitis: a randomized controlled clinical trial. J Clin Periodontol 2017;44:717–28.

41. Trombelli L, Schincaglia G, Checchi L, et al. Combined guided tissue regeneration, root conditioning, and fibrin-fibronectin system application in the treatment of gingival recession. A 15-case report. J Periodontol 1994;65:796–803.
42. Caffesse RG, De LaRosa M, Garza M, et al. Citric acid demineralization and subepithelial connective tissue grafts. J Periodontol 2000;71:568–72.
43. Kassab MM, Cohen RE, Andreana S, et al. The effect of EDTA in attachment gain and root coverage. Compend Contin Educ Dent 2006;27:353–60, quiz 361.
44. Bittencourt S, Ribeiro Edel P, Sallum EA, et al. Root surface biomodification with EDTA for the treatment of gingival recession with a semilunar coronally repositioned flap. J Periodontol 2007;78:1695–701.
45. Zucchelli G, Mounssif I, Stefanini M, et al. Hand and ultrasonic instrumentation in combination with root-coverage surgery: a comparative controlled randomized clinical trial. J Periodontol 2009;80:577–85.
46. Pini Prato G, Rotundo R, Franceschi D, et al. Fourteen-year outcomes of coronally advanced flap for root coverage: follow-up from a randomized trial. J Clin Periodontol 2011;38:715–20.
47. Pini-Prato G, Baldi C, Pagliaro U, et al. Coronally advanced flap procedure for root coverage. Treatment of root surface: root planning versus polishing. J Periodontol 1999;70:1064–76.
48. Dilsiz A, Aydin T, Canakci V, et al. Root surface biomodification with Nd:YAG laser for the treatment of gingival recession with subepithelial connective tissue grafts. Photomed Laser Surg 2010;28:337–43.
49. Dilsiz A, Aydin T, Yavuz MS. Root surface biomodification with an Er:YAG laser for the treatment of gingival recession with subepithelial connective tissue grafts. Photomed Laser Surg 2010;28:511–7.
50. Poormoradi B, Torkzaban P, Gholami L, et al. Effect of Er,Cr (YSGG laser root conditioning on the success of root coverage with subepithelial connective tissue graft): a randomized clinical trial with a 6-month follow-up. J Dent (Tehran) 2018;15:230–9.
51. Damante CA, Karam P, Ferreira R, et al. Root surface demineralization by citric acid/tetracycline gel and aPDT associated to subepithelial connective tissue graft improves root coverage outcomes. A 12-month preliminary randomized clinical trial. J Photochem Photobiol B, Biol 2019;197:111528.
52. McGuire MK, Scheyer ET, Gwaltney C. Commentary: incorporating patient-reported outcomes in periodontal clinical trials. J Periodontol 2014;85:1313–9.
53. Mercieca-Bebber R, King MT, Calvert MJ, et al. The importance of patient-reported outcomes in clinical trials and strategies for future optimization. Patient Relat Outcome Meas 2018;9:353–67.
54. O'Dowd LK, Durham J, McCracken GI, et al. Patients' experiences of the impact of periodontal disease. J Clin Periodontol 2010;37:334–9.
55. Sharma P, Yonel Z, Busby M, et al. Association between periodontal health status and patient-reported outcomes in patients managed in a non-specialist, general dental practice. J Clin Periodontol 2018;45:1440–7.
56. Baiju RM, Peter E, Varghese NO, et al. Patient reported outcome assessment of periodontal therapy: a systematic review. J Clin Diagn Res 2017;11:Zc14–9.
57. Mittal H, John MT, Sekulić S, et al. Patient-reported outcome measures for adult dental patients: a systematic review. J Evid Based Dent Pract 2019;19:53–70.
58. Roman A, Soancă A, Kasaj A, et al. Subepithelial connective tissue graft with or without enamel matrix derivative for the treatment of Miller class I and II gingival recessions: a controlled randomized clinical trial. J Periodontal Res 2013;48(5): 563–72.

Inflammation and Periodontal Regeneration

Hatice Hasturk, DDS, PhD

KEYWORDS

- Inflammation • Periodontal regeneration • Periodontitis • Alveolar bone • Stem cells
- Biologicals

KEY POINTS

- Inflammation is a complex reaction to irritants or harmful agents such as allergens, chemical agents, bacteria, or viruses and it includes vascular and cellular responses, primarily migration and activation of leukocytes from the venous capillary to the injury site starting as an acute reaction.
- If it persists, acute inflammation progresses into a chronic inflammation associated with lymphocyte and macrophage infiltration, blood vessel proliferation, and fibrosis and extends over a longer time and may cause morbidity or mortality in certain conditions.
- If uncontrolled, chronic inflammation leads to continuous tissue (both soft and hard tissue) destruction and ultimately loss of function or organ.
- In periodontal disease, fundamentally, lost periodontal tissues and function due to the chronic disease cannot be rebuilt with traditional periodontal therapies.
- A new avenue of therapeutic approach called "host-modulation therapy" is capable of modulating inflammatory response at multiple levels and offers a new direction in the regeneration of periodontal tissues.
- Specialized proresolution lipid meditators including lipoxin, resolvins, protectins, and maresins are highly promising endogenous molecules modulating the host response during wound healing that promote periodontal tissue regeneration.

INTRODUCTION

Periodontal disease results from a series of pathologic processes affecting the periodontium, including gingiva, periodontal ligament, cementum, and alveolar bone, ultimately leading to tooth loss, functional and esthetic complications.[1] There are various subsets of this disease, the most prevalent of which are gingivitis and periodontitis.[2] Periodontal disease is a complex condition; since it was first described, many etiologic models have been proposed to characterize the disease and its progression appropriately.[3,4] As a result, several classifications have been used to refer

The Forsyth Institute, 245 First Street, Suite 1757, Cambridge, MA 02142, USA
E-mail address: hhasturk@forsyth.org

Dent Clin N Am 66 (2022) 39–51
https://doi.org/10.1016/j.cden.2021.08.003
0011-8532/22/© 2021 Elsevier Inc. All rights reserved.

to periodontal disease and its subsets.[2,5] Periodontal disease is now recognized as a chronic oral inflammatory condition initiated by multiple oral microbial species and associated with a systemic inflammatory state.[6]

The current pathogenesis model of periodontitis has a multilevel framework and is defined by bacterial components, environmental factors, and host and genetic variations.[7] In contrast to previous models, this new framework incorporates genetic variations and environmental factors in the dynamic nature of disease-initiating/resolving biochemical processes to account for the patient-to-patient variations in clinical expression or the site-to-site variations within the same patient. However, the most fundamental controversy in the pathogenesis of periodontal disease is the relationship between microbial biofilm and host immune-inflammatory response. Earlier studies focusing on periodontal biofilm, its composition, and species-level information led the field to the development of preventive and therapeutic modalities based on biofilm removal or resective surgical approaches targeting environmental modifications to, once again, prevent biofilm reinstitution.[8–10] However, although it has been established that the primary etiologic basis for periodontal disease is bacterial, disease progression results from the inadequate resolution of the host's acute inflammatory response to these microbial agents.[11] As a result, a state of chronic inflammation ensues and is itself responsible for the bone and tissue damage observed in patients with periodontitis.[12] Evidence that the host inflammatory response changes the composition of the biofilm, selective for specific organisms[13,14] has not only resulted in a shift in focus of etiologic factors but also changed the understanding of the composition and the role of microbiological species in host-bacteria interaction. Current evidence suggests that *Porphyromonas gingivalis* is a keystone bacterium that causes dysbiosis, defined as significant shifts in the microbiome. The implication that organisms such as *P gingivalis* and *Tannerella forsythia* can cause dysbiosis in the microbiome due to inflammation raises a fundamental question regarding the treatment of periodontitis.[14–18]

TREATMENT OF PERIODONTAL DISEASES: THE UNCHANGED STORY OF A PROGRESSIVE INFLAMMATORY DISEASE

Therapeutic approaches to periodontitis, in a broader aspect, fall under 2 main categories: anti-infective and regenerative therapy. Although anti-infective therapy aims to remove etiologic factors to stop disease progression, regenerative treatments combine anti-infective approaches with procedures aiming to restore the periodontal structures destroyed by the disease. However, both treatment modalities must include maintenance procedures for sustainable efficacy.[19]

The current and, in fact, historical "gold standard" anti-infective and "regenerative" periodontal treatment is scaling and root planing (SRP),[20] which aims to disrupt the biofilm-associated with disease etiology[21] and create a new environment for connective tissue reattachment.[19] Several studies have validated the beneficial effects of SRP combined with personal plaque control.[22–29] SRP has been shown to decrease clinical inflammation, result in microbial shifts to a less pathogenic subgingival flora, reduce pocket depth, improve clinical attachment levels, and halt or slow disease progression.[30,31] However, studies also showed that SRP alone might not be sufficient to eliminate the periodontal pocket presenting a considerable risk of recolonization by the pathogenic bacteria and continuation or progression of the disease.[32] Most importantly, the reattachment without bone gain obtained by scaling and root planing procedure on the disinfected root surfaces is not long-term and can result in pocket reformation as a result of deattachment as early as 3 months following SRP.[33] Surgical procedures that primarily provide access to the site of destruction are often required in patients whose periodontal status remains unimproved after SRP and have been used to treat chronic periodontitis for decades.[19] The rationale for the use of surgery in periodontal treatment is based on its ability to provide better access for removal of etiologic factors, decrease deep probing depths, and regenerate or reconstruct lost periodontal tissues.[34–36] However, the only advantage of surgical approaches without specific procedures designed to regenerate periodontal tissues, including the periodontal ligament and alveolar bone, is its ability to increase the efficacy of root debridement, especially at sites with deep probing depths or bifurcations.[37–47] Both nonsurgical and surgical procedures frequently result in the formation of long junctional epithelium without bone formation or new connective tissue attachment, which is considered weak and unstable.[48,49] Conversely, these procedures may cause a decrease in bone height or gingival recession, leading to esthetic and functional concerns.[40,50]

Adjunct therapies to nonsurgical and surgical approaches have also been proposed and used to overcome the limitation of these mechanical procedures. In this context, several pharmacotherapeutics, including locally administered antimicrobials such as tetracycline, metronidazole, chlorhexidine, doxycycline, and minocycline, have since then been successfully used in periodontal therapy.[51] Local drug delivery as a monotherapy does not provide a superior result when compared with SRP. This approach is practical when used adjunct to SRP, especially in sites that do not respond to conventional therapy. However, the studies conducted with systemic or local antimicrobials revealed that the long epithelial attachment obtained by these treatments is still at high risk of demolishing and pocket formation and biofilm recolonization, especially in susceptible individuals.[50]

Fundamentally, periodontitis is irreversible with the progressive destruction of soft and hard tissues, including bone. Once the periodontal tissues are lost, the healthy periodontal architecture could not be rebuilt.[49] Wound healing is a dynamic process that involves many aspects that are unpredictable and can be challenging following treatment. To date, wound management was the center of the new techniques and treatments to overcome those challenges. Following surgical debridement, the wound healing process takes place with 4 distinct but overlapping phases in sequence involving various cell types, extracellular matrix, cytokines, and growth factors,[52] hemostasis and coagulation (blot clot), inflammation, cell proliferation and migration (fibroblasts and collagen), and remodeling.[53] It is essential to understand wound healing concerning various aspects of cells, molecules, and their functional properties to regenerate tissue functionally and structurally indistinguishable from the original tissue instead of repair that presents fibrotic scars.[54] Under normal conditions, upon injury or surgical debridement, blood clot formation is followed by the initial inflammation, where polymorphonuclear neutrophils and monocytes are activated for efficient phagocytosis and wound debridement by eliminating necrotic tissues. The initial inflammatory response shifts to a late inflammatory phase in which macrophages migrate to the wound area with secreted cytokines or growth factors that promote the wound healing process. Granulation tissue formation is then initiated with collagen accumulation following the inflammatory stage, where cytokines and growth factors induce the migration and proliferation of fibroblasts and endothelial cells into the wound site. The formation and maturation of a new collagen-rich matrix with endothelial cells involving in angiogenesis for revascularization are then activated by this cell-rich granulation tissue.[55] The fate of the granulation tissue maturation is determined by the essential factors, including available functional cells and receptor-mediated events or signals making distinct outcomes, "tissue regeneration" or "repair." Studies with the fetal wounds where scarless and rapid healing occurs[56] have highlighted the importance of proinflammatory and anti-inflammatory cytokine balance and the timely secretion of the growth factors by the cells, and a wound healing process orchestrated by highly specialized resolution molecules and pathways. However, this coordination is affected by several factors in adult tissues[57] with changes in inflammatory response capacity and in oral tissues that continuously face bacterial and physical insults.

In the late 1980 early 90s, a novel surgical approach, namely "guided tissue regeneration (GTR)," was introduced as an alternative to nonsurgical or resective surgical techniques in interproximal areas with vertical or angular bone loss such as class II furcation defects.[58,59] This novel approach was based on the biological concepts of periodontal cellular structures, including fibroblasts, periodontal ligament cells, cementoblasts, and osteoblasts, and their complex interactions. Introducing a physical barrier over the bony defect to prevent the early and rapid down-migration of epithelial cells provided opportunity and time for connective tissue fibroblasts, the periodontal ligament cells, cementoblasts, and alveolar bone cells to migrate to the disinfected and freshly wounded area by mechanical treatment, to initiate a periodontal regenerative wound healing. This approach was the first to result in new bone formation and new tissue attachment that comprises all essential tissue compartments of the periodontium.[60] The ultimate goal was to create a preserved space perfectly sealed from the outside environment, including microbial species. Initially, periodontal regeneration has focused predominantly on bone substitutes and/or barrier membranes to maintain the space and repopulate the cells responsible for defect fill. Within this context, numerous studies testing different bone substitute materials, physical barriers as occluding membranes, root cementum conditioning, and combination of these with adjunct use of systemic and local antibiotics for adjunctive antimicrobial therapies, have reported varying levels of success and failures over the last 30 years since the concept was first introduced.[61] Systematic reviews on regenerative periodontal treatments show evidence that GTR has a more significant effect on improved attachment gain, reduced pocket depth, more gain in hard tissue with only a minor increase in gingival recession than open flap debridement.[62] However, they also highlight marked variability between studies and the clinical relevance of these changes that is unknown.[63]

Thus, today the treatment of periodontitis in the regeneration of lost tissues, including gingiva, periodontal ligament, cementum, and alveolar bone, is still challenging with unpredictable outcomes and at under the desirable levels, or significant side effects hinder their success.[64] Most importantly, as chronic adult periodontitis often results in horizontal bone loss around the teeth, supra alveolar bone growth on denuded root surfaces has not yet been achieved with any of the therapeutic approaches, which requires a combination of tissue engineering, biologicals, and immune modulation with specifically targeted pathways and molecules that drive tissue formation.

HOST MODULATORY THERAPIES DIRECTED AT THE REGENERATION OF THE PERIODONTIUM

As described in the previous section, the classical "GTR" promotes the critical cell and tissue compartments to regenerate lost tissues under a guided strategy. It is in theory, and in rare instances, it accomplishes the goal of the treatment with a complete regeneration. However, this is not only a rare event; it is also unpredictable, and many factors including flap design, space, type of materials used, location of the tooth, defect size, number of defect walls remained, pulp vitality, patient's age, smoking, and medical conditions such as diabetes mellitus could influence it.[65]

More recently, several technologies, including growth factors, biologicals, and scaffolds, have evolved to be viewed as emerging therapeutic approaches for periodontal regeneration.[62] In attempts to promote certain cell types for proliferation or tissue formation, several biologicals, including growth factors, collagen, platelet-rich plasma (PRP), plasma rich growth factor (PRGF), fibrin sealant, have been used with varying capacities in regenerating periodontal tissues lost to the disease.[66–68] Among these approaches, enamel matrix derivates (EMDs) have been used extensively in periodontal regeneration in vertical interproximal defects or furcation involvements.[69] EMD is considered a tissue healing agent derived from proteins during cementogenesis in tooth development to enrich the cellular layers and stimulate tissue regeneration around teeth. Amelogenin is the main protein of EMD known to inhibit epithelial growth, which is the key component of the GTR strategy. In addition, amelogenin has been shown to exert osteoprotective properties and anti-inflammatory actions that enhance soft tissue healing.[70] Furthermore, several in-vivo and in vitro studies have shown EMD's role on cytokine balance by reducing the secretion of chemokines and proinflammatory cytokines, providing a smooth transition to hemostasis and complete healing.[71]

PRP and PRGF are autologous bioactive substances that contain biologically active proteins which bind to the fibrin mesh or extracellular matrix, promoting the recruitment of stem cells and wound healing. However, although these factors have been proven to promote tissue healing and bone formation in extraction sockets, sinus augmentation, and around dental implants,[62] their use in periodontal defects and capabilities of promoting periodontal regenerations are limited.

Recent consensus reports[72,73] reviewed the current FDA-approved and nonapproved emerging therapeutic approaches focusing on host modulation and tissue engineering such as protein and peptide therapy,[74] cell-based therapy,[75] scaffolds,[76] bone anabolics, and lasers. FDA-approved products evaluated included EMD; recombinant human platelet-derived growth factor; and an anorganic bone matrix, whereas nonapproved therapeutic modalities included recombinant human fibroblast growth factor-2; recombinant human growth differentiation factor-5; bone morphogenetic proteins (BMP-2, BMP-7, BMP-6, and BMP-12); parathyroid hormone/teriparatide; brain-derived neurotrophic factor; and sclerostin antibodies.[77] Mesenchymal stem cells, bone marrow stromal cells, periodontal ligament cells, embryonic stem cells, and induced pluripotent stem cells[78] were reviewed among cell-based therapeutic approaches, viral and nonviral vectors as genetic therapies and scaffolds[79] that show promising results for delivery of growth factors and gene therapy and combination of either natural or synthetic polymeric materials in periodontal regeneration. However, although these therapies appear viable as emerging regenerative approaches for periodontal hard and soft tissue regeneration with the potential of reconstructing the entire periodontium, the cost-to-benefit ratio and safety issues still need to be overcome, and most importantly, there is insufficient evidence with those therapies to warrant definitive clinical recommendations.[73]

HOST MODULATION THERAPIES DIRECTED AT RESOLUTION OF INFLAMMATION IN REGENERATIVE PERIODONTAL TREATMENT

In the event of uncontrolled host defense mechanisms, tissue engineering, regeneration, and reconstruction of both diseased and injured tissues are significantly hampered.[80] Inflammation is a host defense mechanism orchestrated by key cellular and molecular events leading to activation of defensive immune subsets to limit detrimental injury, eliminate pathogenic agents, and remove infected cells. Under normal conditions, a parallel host mechanism operates to contain inflammatory response leading to health or stability.[81] Thus, resolution of inflammation is an effective suspension on the proinflammatory pathways to avoid the tissue damage inside the host and leads to the reestablishment of tissue homeostasis. However, uncontrolled inflammation may cause tissue damage by perturbing homeostasis toward immune dysregulation and chronic inflammation. Dysregulation of the resolution pathways can negatively impact tissue functionality and contribute to the disease state.

In contaminated traumatic wounds involving bone, an uncontrolled inflammatory response causes neutrophil-mediated tissue injury that, in turn, leads to irreversible bone loss. Neutrophils are essential in microbial host defense, but chronic neutrophil activation, due to failure of a timely switch from inflammatory to resolution pathways, can release noxious materials leading to host tissue injury and loss of function.[82] Likewise, in chronic osteolytic inflammatory diseases such as periodontitis,[83,84] a failure of endogenous resolution pathways and removal of microbial challenge result in tissue destruction.[85] Therefore, one of the most crucial elements determining the fate of the wound healing process and success of the regeneration is the inflammatory response to the treatment and endogenous anti-inflammatory, and proresolving mechanisms that activate wound healing with tissue regeneration instead of fibrosis and scarring[86,87] are crucial.

Modulation of inflammatory response and control of inflammation is, however, a challenging issue. To this end, anti-inflammatory agents such as nonsteroidal anti-inflammatory drugs (NSAIDs), although logical, do not provide predictable outcomes, partly due to side effects and compliance issues.[88] In addition, anti-inflammatory agents can downregulate essential immune cell functions critical for wound healing; therefore, they could be toxic to regeneration.[89]

The discovery of the new families of lipoxins, EPA- and DHA-derived chemical mediators, namely resolvins and protectins, open new avenues to design resolution-targeted therapies to control unwanted side-effects of aberrant inflammation.[90] The findings of series of preclinical in vitro[91–94] and in vivo[14,95,96] studies demonstrated the beneficial role of the lipid mediators in temporal resolution of inflammation and returned to hemostasis in experimental periodontitis. Mediators of resolution of inflammation also have actions beyond the control of neutrophils; modulation of osteoclast and osteoblast function in a receptor-mediated fashion in wound healing and bone regeneration.[97,98] Furthermore, exciting findings with animal models proved an old hypothesis known as "self-healing capacity if promoted" and revealed that endogenous control of inflammation directly impacts bone healing and regeneration.[14,95] Studies with lipoxin and resolvins in experimental periodontitis in mice, rats, and rabbits demonstrated that specialized proresolution lipid mediators (SMPs) resolve the inflammation and promote regeneration of soft and hard tissues around teeth.[99] Furthermore, benzo lipoxin A4 (a stable analog of lipoxin A4) resulted in a complete periodontal regeneration with the periodontal ligament, new cementum, and alveolar bone formation in chronic periodontal defects compared to conventional flap surgery.[15]

The incorporation of proresolving mediators into nanoparticles constructed from natural microparticles has proven to be a practical approach for promoting survival in animal models of sepsis[100] and reducing inflammation and stimulating resolution.[101] Using this "proresolving nanomedicine" approach, a recent study demonstrated that complete regeneration of soft and hard tissues lost to inflammatory periodontal disease in a large animal model mimicking human periodontal disease and wound healing process following surgical debridement was clinically possible[15] (Fig. 1). Furthermore, this approach not only resulted in a resolution of inflammation at the local wound but

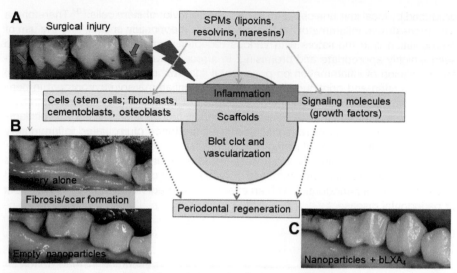

Fig. 1. Schematic illustration of regulation of inflammatory response by specialized proresolving lipid mediators in the periodontal regenerative treatment in a minipig model of chronic periodontitis. (*A*) Injury upon surgical debridement leading to bleeding and subsequent blot clot formation followed by early inflammatory response by neutrophils and late inflammatory response by macrophages. (*B*) Treatment of periodontal defect by surgical debridement and granulation tissue removal results in fibrosis/scar formation without regenerative procedure. (*C*) Modulation of inflammation by specialized proresolving lipid mediators (ie, lipoxin A4) acting through receptor-mediated events over the targeted cells promoting secretion of signaling molecules to induce an orchestrated tissue healing along with the use of scaffolds (ie, nanoparticles) that maintains the space and timely releases the proinflammatory mediators to the environment results in the regeneration without fibrosis/scar formation.

also promoted systemic endogenous biosynthesis of SPMs and dampened production of proinflammatory mediators, indicating that nanoparticles constructed with the stable lipoxin analog, benzo-lipoxin A4 (bLXA4) potentiates the anabolic actions of bLXA4[102] in the regeneration of tissues lost to inflammatory disease by activating distinct proresolving and tissue-protective pathways.[15] Currently, bLXA4 is in the process of drug development to treat periodontal diseases (ClinicalTrials.gov NCT02342691).

NEW AVENUES IN THE REGENERATION OF PERIODONTAL TISSUES

For the last decade, the concept of stem cells and their role in the regeneration of periodontium has become the center of attention in periodontal medicine. Viable and highly promising findings opened up the possibility of a new therapeutic approach in periodontal regeneration with the increase of knowledge on the actions of stem cells and technological advancements.[103] However, as briefly mentioned in the previous sections, several areas need to be improved, such as developing appropriate scaffolds that deliver the cells and growth factors even in the infective healing environment and promote resolution of inflammation returning homeostasis. Furthermore, it is demonstrated that even with well-designed tissue engineering techniques, inflammation remains a "demon" that needs to be controlled and modulated.[15,73] Once an inflammatory response has been initiated, cytokines, interferons, and other mediators produced by local immune cells can impact the behavior of stem cells.[104] Therefore, a well-orchestrated inflammatory response seems exceptionally critical, and the use of proresolution lipid mediators with various receptor-mediated actions in that sense seems highly appropriate and promising. In a recent study, the impact of activation and resolution of inflammation on periodontal ligament stem cells, which are critical for regeneration and continuously exposed to an inflammatory environment in periodontal tissues, has been investigated in vitro.[105] SPMs (maresins, resolvins) strongly impacted the restoration of stem cells' regenerative functions exposed to a proinflammatory imbalance. This work highlighted the importance of regulated inflammatory response on cells capable of giving rise to the tissues that comprise the entire periodontium. These promising developments in the regeneration of periodontal tissues open up a new direction with immense potential to the clinical translation that could power the field of periodontics with an effective and predictable tool in the treatment of periodontal disease.

CLINICS CARE POINTS

Periodontal regeneration is the ultimate goal of periodontal treatment, but several key factors can influence the desired outcome. Based on the information in this article, the following key points should be considered for achieving periodontal regeneration. These include:

- A detailed patient medical history.
- Removal of microbial plaque and calculus and a successful home care.
- Control of independent risk factors, such as smoking, medical conditions (eg, diabetes).
- Use of techniques to maintain space, blood clot and manipulation of soft tissue for primary closure.
- Use of biologicals, scaffolds, or cells that have potential of promoting wound healing, stability of blood clot and bone formation.
- Use of compounds that are capable of promoting resolution of inflammation instead of blocking inflammation.

DISCLOSURE

Dr Hasturk is inventor of several granted and pending licensed and unlicensed patents awarded to the Forsyth Institute that are subject to royalty payments. Dr Hasturk received funding from NIDCR grant R01-DE025020.

REFERENCES

1. Kinane DF. Causation and pathogenesis of periodontal disease. Periodontol 2000 2001;25:8–20.
2. Armitage GC. Development of a classification system for periodontal diseases and conditions. Ann Periodontol 1999;4(1):1–6.
3. Genco RJ, Borgnakke WS. Risk factors for periodontal disease. Periodontol 2000 2013;62(1):59–94.
4. Kinane DF, Stathopoulou PG, Papapanou PN. Periodontal diseases. Nat Rev Dis Primers 2017;3:17038.
5. Papapanou PN, Sanz M, Buduneli N, et al. Periodontitis: consensus report of workgroup 2 of the 2017 World Workshop on the classification of periodontal

and peri-implant diseases and conditions. J Periodontol 2018;89(Suppl 1): S173–82.

6. Loos BG, Van Dyke TE. The role of inflammation and genetics in periodontal disease. Periodontol 2000 2020;83(1):26–39.

7. Bartold PM, Van Dyke TE. Periodontitis: a host-mediated disruption of microbial homeostasis. Unlearning learned concepts. Periodontol 2000 2013;62(1): 203–17.

8. Anerud A, Loe H, Boysen H, et al. The natural history of periodontal disease in man. Changes in gingival health and oral hygiene before 40 years of age. J Periodontal Res 1979;14(6):526–40.

9. Loe H, Anerud A, Boysen H, et al. The natural history of periodontal disease in man. The rate of periodontal destruction before 40 years of age. J Periodontol 1978;49(12):607–20.

10. Kuramitsu HK, He X, Lux R, et al. Interspecies interactions within oral microbial communities. Microbiol Mol Biol Rev 2007;71(4):653–70.

11. Van Dyke TE. The management of inflammation in periodontal disease. J Periodontol 2008;79(8 Suppl):1601–8.

12. Serhan CN. Novel omega – 3-derived local mediators in anti-inflammation and resolution. Pharmacol Ther 2005;105(1):7–21.

13. Finlay BB, Medzhitov R. Host-microbe interactions: fulfilling a niche. Cell Host Microbe 2007;1(1):3–4.

14. Hasturk H, Kantarci A, Goguet-Surmenian E, et al. Resolvin E1 regulates inflammation at the cellular and tissue level and restores tissue homeostasis in vivo. J Immunol 2007;179(10):7021–9.

15. Van Dyke TE, Hasturk H, Kantarci A, et al. Proresolving nanomedicines activate bone regeneration in periodontitis. J Dent Res 2015;94(1):148–56.

16. Darveau RP. Periodontitis: a polymicrobial disruption of host homeostasis. Nat Rev Microbiol 2010;8(7):481–90.

17. Hajishengallis G, Liang S, Payne MA, et al. Low-abundance biofilm species orchestrates inflammatory periodontal disease through the commensal microbiota and complement. Cell Host Microbe 2011;10(5):497–506.

18. Hajishengallis G, Lamont RJ. Beyond the red complex and into more complexity: the polymicrobial synergy and dysbiosis (PSD) model of periodontal disease etiology. Mol Oral Microbiol 2012;27(6):409–19.

19. Treatment of plaque-induced gingivitis, chronic periodontitis, and other clinical conditions. J Periodontol 2001;72(12):1790–800.

20. Cobb CM. Clinical significance of non-surgical periodontal therapy: an evidence-based perspective of scaling and root planing. J Clin Periodontol 2002;29(Suppl 2):6–16.

21. Socransky SS, Haffajee AD. Dental biofilms: difficult therapeutic targets. Periodontol 2000 2002;28:12–55.

22. Morrison EC, Ramfjord SP, Hill RW. Short-term effects of initial, nonsurgical periodontal treatment (hygienic phase). J Clin Periodontol 1980;7(3):199–211.

23. Garrett JS. Effects of nonsurgical periodontal therapy on periodontitis in humans. A review. J Clin Periodontol 1983;10(5):515–23.

24. Badersten A, Nilveus R, Egelberg J. Effect of nonsurgical periodontal therapy. I. Moderately advanced periodontitis. J Clin Periodontol 1981;8(1):57–72.

25. Badersten A, Nilveus R, Egelberg J. Effect of nonsurgical periodontal therapy. III. Single versus repeated instrumentation. J Clin Periodontol 1984;11(2): 114–24.

26. Badersten A, Nilveus R, Egelberg J. Effect of nonsurgical periodontal therapy. II. Severely advanced periodontitis. J Clin Periodontol 1984;11(1):63–76.

27. Hughes TP, Caffesse RG. Gingival changes following scaling, root planning and oral hygiene. A biometric evaluation. J Periodontol 1978;49(5):245–52.

28. Magnusson I, Lindhe J, Yoneyama T, et al. Recolonization of a subgingival microbiota following scaling in deep pockets. J Clin Periodontol 1984;11(3): 193–207.

29. Mousques T, Listgarten MA, Phillips RW. Effect of scaling and root planing on the composition of the human subgingival microbial flora. J Periodontal Res 1980;15(2):144–51.

30. Drisko CH. Nonsurgical periodontal therapy. Periodontol 2000 2001;25:77–88.

31. Van der Weijden GAF, Dekkers GJ, Slot DE. Success of non-surgical periodontal therapy in adult periodontitis patients: a retrospective analysis. Int J Dent Hyg 2019;17(4):309–17.

32. Mombelli A. Microbial colonization of the periodontal pocket and its significance for periodontal therapy. Periodontol 2000 2018;76(1):85–96.

33. Sculean A, Windisch P, Keglevich T, et al. Histologic evaluation of human intrabony defects following non-surgical periodontal therapy with and without application of an enamel matrix protein derivative. J Periodontol 2003;74(2):153–60.

34. Consensus report. Surgical pocket therapy. Ann Periodontol 1996;1(1):618–20.

35. Consensus report. Periodontal regeneration around natural teeth. Ann Periodontol 1996;1(1):667–70.

36. Consensus report. Mucogingival therapy. Ann Periodontol 1996;1(1):702–6.

37. Pihlstrom BL, McHugh RB, Oliphant TH, et al. Comparison of surgical and nonsurgical treatment of periodontal disease. A review of current studies and additional results after 6 1/2 years. J Clin Periodontol 1983;10(5):524–41.

38. Hill RW, Ramfjord SP, Morrison EC, et al. Four types of periodontal treatment compared over two years. J Periodontol 1981;52(11):655–62.

39. Kaldahl WB, Kalkwarf KL, Patil KD, et al. Evaluation of four modalities of periodontal therapy. Mean probing depth, probing attachment level and recession changes. J Periodontol 1988;59(12):783–93.

40. Kaldahl WB, Kalkwarf KL, Patil KD, et al. Long-term evaluation of periodontal therapy: I. Response to 4 therapeutic modalities. J Periodontol 1996;67(2): 93–102.

41. Becker W, Becker BE, Ochsenbein C, et al. A longitudinal study comparing scaling, osseous surgery and modified Widman procedures. Results after one year. J Periodontol 1988;59(6):351–65.

42. Ramfjord SP, Caffesse RG, Morrison EC, et al. 4 modalities of periodontal treatment compared over 5 years. J Clin Periodontol 1987;14(8):445–52.

43. Antczak-Bouckoms A, Joshipura K, Burdick E, et al. Meta-analysis of surgical versus non-surgical methods of treatment for periodontal disease. J Clin Periodontol 1993;20(4):259–68.

44. Pihlstrom BL, Oliphant TH, McHugh RB. Molar and nonmolar teeth compared over 6 1/2 years following two methods of periodontal therapy. J Periodontol 1984;55(9):499–504.

45. Lindhe J, Westfelt E, Nyman S, et al. Healing following surgical/non-surgical treatment of periodontal disease. A clinical study. J Clin Periodontol 1982; 9(2):115–28.

46. Caffesse RG, Sweeney PL, Smith BA. Scaling and root planing with and without periodontal flap surgery. J Clin Periodontol 1986;13(3):205–10.

47. Buchanan SA, Robertson PB. Calculus removal by scaling/root planing with and without surgical access. J Periodontol 1987;58(3):159–63.
48. Caton J, Nyman S. Histometric evaluation of periodontal surgery. I. The modified Widman flap procedure. J Clin Periodontol 1980;7(3):212–23.
49. Caton J, Nyman S, Zander H. Histometric evaluation of periodontal surgery. II. Connective tissue attachment levels after four regenerative procedures. J Clin Periodontol 1980;7(3):224–31.
50. Goodson JM, Haffajee AD, Socransky SS, et al. Control of periodontal infections: a randomized controlled trial I. The primary outcome attachment gain and pocket depth reduction at treated sites. J Clin Periodontol 2012;39(6):526–36.
51. Williams RC. Understanding and managing periodontal diseases: a notable past, a promising future. J Periodontol 2008;79(8 Suppl):1552–9.
52. Cho YD, Kim WJ, Ryoo HM, et al. Current advances of epigenetics in periodontology from ENCODE project: a review and future perspectives. Clin Epigenetics 2021;13(1):92.
53. Polimeni G, Xiropaidis AV, Wikesjo UM. Biology and principles of periodontal wound healing/regeneration. Periodontol 2000 2006;41:30–47.
54. Nikoloudaki G, Creber K, Hamilton DW. Wound healing and fibrosis: a contrasting role for periostin in skin and the oral mucosa. Am J Physiol Cell Physiol 2020; 318(6):C1065–77.
55. Susin C, Fiorini T, Lee J, et al. Wound healing following surgical and regenerative periodontal therapy. Periodontol 2000 2015;68(1):83–98.
56. Moore AL, Marshall CD, Barnes LA, et al. Scarless wound healing: transitioning from fetal research to regenerative healing. Wiley Interdiscip Rev Dev Biol 2018;7(2).
57. Leavitt T, Hu MS, Marshall CD, et al. Scarless wound healing: finding the right cells and signals. Cell Tissue Res 2016;365(3):483–93.
58. Gottlow J, Nyman S, Lindhe J, et al. New attachment formation in the human periodontium by guided tissue regeneration. Case reports. J Clin Periodontol 1986;13(6):604–16.
59. Karring T, Nyman S, Gottlow J, et al. Development of the biological concept of guided tissue regeneration–animal and human studies. Periodontol 2000 1993; 1(1):26–35.
60. McCulloch CA. Basic considerations in periodontal wound healing to achieve regeneration. Periodontol 2000 1993;1(1):16–25.
61. Wang HL, Greenwell H, Fiorellini J, et al. Periodontal regeneration. J Periodontol 2005;76(9):1601–22.
62. Mancini L, Romandini M, Fratini A, et al. Biomaterials for periodontal and peri-implant regeneration. Materials (Basel) 2021;14(12):3319.
63. Needleman IG, Worthington HV, Giedrys-Leeper E, et al. Guided tissue regeneration for periodontal infra-bony defects. Cochrane Database Syst Rev 2006;(2):CD001724.
64. Chen FM, Shelton RM, Jin Y, et al. Localized delivery of growth factors for periodontal tissue regeneration: role, strategies, and perspectives. Med Res Rev 2009;29(3):472–513.
65. Reynolds MA, Kao RT, Camargo PM, et al. Periodontal regeneration - intrabony defects: a consensus report from the AAP Regeneration Workshop. J Periodontol 2015;86(2 Suppl):S105–7.
66. Esposito M, Grusovin MG, Papanikolaou N, et al. Enamel matrix derivative (Emdogain(R)) for periodontal tissue regeneration in intrabony defects. Cochrane Database Syst Rev 2009;(4):CD003875.

67. Darby IB, Morris KH. A systematic review of the use of growth factors in human periodontal regeneration. J Periodontol 2013;84(4):465–76.
68. Murakami S. Periodontal tissue regeneration by signaling molecule(s): what role does basic fibroblast growth factor (FGF-2) have in periodontal therapy? Periodontol 2000 2011;56(1):188–208.
69. Miron RJ, Sculean A, Cochran DL, et al. Twenty years of enamel matrix derivative: the past, the present and the future. J Clin Periodontol 2016;43(8):668–83.
70. Durstberger G, Nguyen PQ, Hohensinner V, et al. Effect of enamel matrix derivatives on osteoclast formation from PBMC of periodontitis patients and healthy individuals after interaction with activated endothelial cells. Medicina (Kaunas) 2021;57(3):269.
71. Zeldich E, Koren R, Dard M, et al. Enamel matrix derivative induces the expression of tissue inhibitor of matrix metalloproteinase-3 in human gingival fibroblasts via extracellular signal-regulated kinase. J Periodontal Res 2010;45(2): 200–6.
72. Sanz M, Dahlin C, Apatzidou D, et al. Biomaterials and regenerative technologies used in bone regeneration in the craniomaxillofacial region: consensus report of group 2 of the 15th European Workshop on Periodontology on Bone Regeneration. J Clin Periodontol 2019;46(Suppl 21):82–91.
73. Cochran DL, Cobb CM, Bashutski JD, et al. Emerging regenerative approaches for periodontal reconstruction: a consensus report from the AAP Regeneration Workshop. J Periodontol 2015;86(2 Suppl):S153–6.
74. Foster BL, Nagatomo KJ, Nociti FH Jr, et al. Central role of pyrophosphate in acellular cementum formation. PLoS One 2012;7(6):e38393.
75. Arany PR, Cho A, Hunt TD, et al. Photoactivation of endogenous latent transforming growth factor-beta1 directs dental stem cell differentiation for regeneration. Sci Transl Med 2014;6(238):238–69.
76. Costa PF, Vaquette C, Zhang Q, et al. Advanced tissue engineering scaffold design for regeneration of the complex hierarchical periodontal structure. J Clin Periodontol 2014;41(3):283–94.
77. Oortgiesen DA, Walboomers XF, Bronckers AL, et al. Periodontal regeneration using an injectable bone cement combined with BMP-2 or FGF-2. J Tissue Eng Regen Med 2014;8(3):202–9.
78. Daigo Y, Daigo E, Fukuoka H, et al. Wound healing and cell dynamics including mesenchymal and dental pulp stem cells induced by photobiomodulation therapy: an example of socket-preserving effects after tooth extraction in rats and a literature review. Int J Mol Sci 2020;21(18):6850.
79. Ivanovski S, Vaquette C, Gronthos S, et al. Multiphasic scaffolds for periodontal tissue engineering. J Dent Res 2014;93(12):1212–21.
80. Lumelsky NL. Commentary: engineering of tissue healing and regeneration. Tissue Eng 2007;13(7):1393–8.
81. Panigrahy D, Gilligan MM, Serhan CN, et al. Resolution of inflammation: an organizing principle in biology and medicine. Pharmacol Ther 2021;107879.
82. Dalli J, Chiang N, Serhan CN. Identification of 14-series sulfido-conjugated mediators that promote resolution of infection and organ protection. Proc Natl Acad Sci U S A 2014;111(44):E4753–61.
83. Offenbacher S, Barros SP, Beck JD. Rethinking periodontal inflammation. J Periodontol 2008;79(8 Suppl):1577–84.
84. Williams RC. Host modulation for the treatment of periodontal disease. Compend Contin Educ Dent 2008;29(3):160–2, 164, 166–168 passim.

85. Hasturk H, Kantarci A, Van Dyke TE. Paradigm shift in the pharmacological management of periodontal diseases. Front Oral Biol 2012;15:160–76.
86. Ortega-Gomez A, Perretti M, Soehnlein O. Resolution of inflammation: an integrated view. EMBO Mol Med 2013;5(5):661–74.
87. Martin CR, Zaman MM, Gilkey C, et al. Resolvin D1 and lipoxin A4 improve alveolarization and normalize septal wall thickness in a neonatal murine model of hyperoxia-induced lung injury. PLoS One 2014;9(6):e98773.
88. Etikala A, Tattan M, Askar H, et al. Effects of NSAIDs on Periodontal and Dental Implant Therapy. Compend Contin Educ Dent 2019;40(2):e1–9.
89. Dalli J. Does promoting resolution instead of inhibiting inflammation represent the new paradigm in treating infections? Mol Aspects Med 2017;58:12–20.
90. Serhan CN, Chiang N, Dalli J. The resolution code of acute inflammation: Novel pro-resolving lipid mediators in resolution. Semin Immunol 2015;27(3):200–15.
91. Mustafa M, Zarrough A, Bolstad AI, et al. Resolvin D1 protects periodontal ligament. Am J Physiol Cell Physiol 2013;305(6):C673–9.
92. Gao L, Faibish D, Fredman G, et al. Resolvin E1 and chemokine-like receptor 1 mediate bone preservation. J Immunol 2013;190(2):689–94.
93. Herrera BS, Kantarci A, Zarrough A, et al. LXA4 actions direct fibroblast function and wound closure. Biochem Biophys Res Commun 2015;464(4):1072–7.
94. Oner F, Alvarez C, Yaghmoor W, et al. Resolvin E1 regulates Th17 function and T cell activation. Front Immunol 2021;12:637983.
95. Hasturk H, Kantarci A, Ohira T, et al. RvE1 protects from local inflammation and osteoclast- mediated bone destruction in periodontitis. FASEB J 2006;20(2): 401–3.
96. Lee CT, Teles R, Kantarci A, et al. Resolvin E1 reverses experimental periodontitis and dysbiosis. J Immunol 2016;197(7):2796–806.
97. Herrera BS, Ohira T, Gao L, et al. An endogenous regulator of inflammation, resolvin E1, modulates osteoclast differentiation and bone resorption. Br J Pharmacol 2008;155(8):1214–23.
98. Zhu M, Van Dyke TE, Gyurko R. Resolvin E1 regulates osteoclast fusion via DC-STAMP and NFATc1. FASEB J 2013;27(8):3344–53.
99. Van Dyke TE. Shifting the paradigm from inhibitors of inflammation to resolvers of inflammation in periodontitis. J Periodontol 2020;91(Suppl 1):S19–25.
100. Dalli J, Norling LV, Montero-Melendez T, et al. Microparticle alpha-2-macroglobulin enhances pro-resolving responses and promotes survival in sepsis. EMBO Mol Med 2014;6(1):27–42.
101. Silver MA, Pick R, Brilla CG, et al. Reactive and reparative fibrillar collagen remodelling in the hypertrophied rat left ventricle: two experimental models of myocardial fibrosis. Cardiovasc Res 1990;24(9):741–7.
102. Yao C, Sakata D, Esaki Y, et al. Prostaglandin E2-EP4 signaling promotes immune inflammation through Th1 cell differentiation and Th17 cell expansion. Nat Med 2009;15(6):633–40.
103. Queiroz A, Albuquerque-Souza E, Gasparoni LM, et al. Therapeutic potential of periodontal ligament stem cells. World J Stem Cells 2021;13(6):605–18.
104. Michael S, Achilleos C, Panayiotou T, et al. Inflammation shapes stem cells and stemness during infection and beyond. Front Cell Dev Biol 2016;4:118.
105. Albuquerque-Souza E, Schulte F, Chen T, et al. Maresin-1 and resolvin E1 promote regenerative properties of periodontal ligament stem cells under inflammatory conditions. Front Immunol 2020;11:585530.

Stem Cell Applications in Periodontal Regeneration

Mark Bartold, BDS, PhD, DDSc, FRACDS(Perio)*, Saso Ivanovski, BDSc, BDentSt, MDSc(Perio), PhD

KEYWORDS

- Periodontal regeneration • Stem cells • Tissue engineering

KEY POINTS

- What are stem cells?
- Dental stem cells for periodontal regeneration.
- Extraoral stem cells for periodontal regeneration.
- Stem cell periodontal regeneration in humans.
- Future use of stem cell-based therapies in periodontal regeneration.

INTRODUCTION

What Is Periodontal Regeneration?

Periodontal regeneration is the full restoration of a damaged periodontal attachment apparatus (cementum, periodontal ligament, and alveolar bone) to its original architecture and function.[1] It is a biological term defined by its histologic characteristics of *restitutio ad integrum* (restoration to original condition) of the periodontal architecture, including new cementum, periodontal ligament, and alveolar bone surrounding a tooth that has been deprived of its attachment apparatus usually because of the effects of periodontitis. Clinically, periodontal regeneration is characterized by a gain in clinical attachment, reduction in pocket depth, and radiographic evidence of an increase in alveolar bone levels. However, these observations cannot distinguish between regeneration and reparative healing, especially when various grafting and "regenerative" techniques have been used. Accordingly, these clinical outcomes should be viewed more as a result of periodontal reconstruction than periodontal regeneration per se. Therefore, periodontal reconstruction is viewed as a clinical term used to coin clinical and radiographic improvements, that is, gains in clinical attachment, reduced probing pocket depth, and bone fill, representing reparative and/or partial regenerative healing.

Currently, periodontal regeneration is recognized as being biologically possible but clinically unpredictable and remains an elusive goal. Successful periodontal

School of Dentistry, University of Queensland, UQ Oral Health Centre (Bldg. 883), 288 Herston Road, Herston, Qld 4006, Australia
* Corresponding author. 1 Milton Avenue, Beaumont, South Australia 5066, Australia.
E-mail address: mark.bartold@adelaide.edu.au

Dent Clin N Am 66 (2022) 53–74
https://doi.org/10.1016/j.cden.2021.06.002
0011-8532/22/© 2021 Elsevier Inc. All rights reserved.

regeneration is best illustrated within the context of the principles of the "number needed to treat" (NNT) principle, a measure used to assess a health care intervention's effectiveness. NNT calculates the average number of patients who need to be treated to prevent one additional poor outcome (ie, the number of patients who need to be treated for benefit compared with a control in a clinical trial).

In a recent systematic review, it was noted that the NNT for the current gold-standard periodontal regeneration technique, guided tissue regeneration (GTR), to obtain one extra intrabony defect achieving pocket depth (PD) ≤3 mm or PD ≤4 mm over papilla preservation flaps (control) was 2 and 4, respectively.[2] Although this is an improvement on previous studies indicating the NNT for GTR to achieve one extra site gaining 2 mm or more attachment over open flap debridement was 8,[3] it is still considered far from ideal.[4] Therefore, research efforts are continuing to explore improved ways to achieve predictable periodontal regeneration. To achieve this, several fundamental concepts must be adhered to. First, to fill a defect with a substance that has no relevance to the next functional state of reconstruction is irrational.[5] Furthermore, it has been long recognized that the dental profession has become obsessed with filling holes in bone rather than studying the natural healing processes required for true periodontal regeneration.[6] Clearly, regenerative treatment of periodontal defects with an agent or procedure requires that each functional stage of reconstruction be grounded in a biologically directed process.[5]

Regeneration of the periodontium mimics periodontal development and requires a very complex spatial and hierarchical sequence of events. Critical to this process is the recruitment of precursor (stem) cells that have the potential to differentiate and produce cementum, periodontal ligament, and alveolar bone.[5] In this context, stem cell–based tissue engineering approaches have provided novel, biologically based avenues for enhancing periodontal regeneration.

In this article, the authors consider the substantial advances that have been made in recent years in stem cell–based periodontal regeneration. These advances include identifying dental- and nondental-derived stem cells with the capacity to facilitate periodontal regeneration, human clinical trials, and emerging concepts, including cell banking, good manufacturing processes, and overall clinical translation.

A CELLULAR APPROACH TO PERIODONTAL REGENERATION

Following the discovery of numerous subsets and subpopulations of cells residing within the periodontal tissues, it became necessary to study these cells in more detail.[7,8] A significant advance was made when it became possible to clone and expand cells from normal, inflamed, and regenerating periodontal tissues.[9,10] These studies provided new avenues of investigations and now pave the way for exciting developments in tissue engineering using cell seeding methodologies, gene manipulation, and fabrication of bio-scaffolds for cell delivery.[5]

WHAT ARE STEM CELLS?

By definition, a stem cell refers to an undifferentiated cell capable of self-renewal and multilineage differentiation.[11] These cells can replicate, producing a pool of stem cells with the potential, under specific conditions (in vivo and in vitro), to differentiate and mature along multiple lineages, resulting in a range of tissue-specific cell phenotypes and morphotypes. Importantly, stem cells have the capacity for prolonged self-renewal and/or differentiation controlled by a myriad of intrinsic mechanisms that, in turn, are regulated by the local niche environment of each stem cell.[12–14]

Three broad categories of stem cells are recognized: (i) embryonic stem cells, (ii) postnatal (adult or somatic) stem cells, and (iii) the genetically modified differentiated cells known as induced pluripotent stem cells (IPSC). Embryonic stem cells have a high pluripotent potential and can differentiate into all 220 types of specialized cells that comprise the human body.[13–15] Because of the ethical issues surrounding the acquisition of embryonic stem cells, their clinical use is limited. To get around this problem, it is possible to genetically manipulate and reprogram somatic cells into cells with an embryonic stem cell phenotype regarding morphology, gene expression profiles, proliferation, and differentiation capacities, but without the ethical concerns of embryonic stem cells.[16–18] Just more than a decade ago, the first reports appeared describing the reprogramming of somatic cells into pluripotent cells with a differentiation and self-renewal capacity comparable to embryonic stem cells.[16] These cells were termed "induced pluripotent stem cells" and are considered to provide an ethically viable alternative to embryonic stem cells in regenerative medicine. However, the genetics required for the generation of IPSC are not without concerns, including the potential induction of tumorigenic properties, raising a significant safety challenge in the use of these cells for regenerative therapies.[19,20]

Adult stem cells are responsible for the regeneration of damaged tissues. Initially, these cells were termed stromal precursor cells, but they have been referred to as mesenchymal stem cells (MSC) in recent times. MSC are present in adult tissues and can differentiate into multiple specialized cell types.[21–26] Their accessibility, high growth capacity, and multipotential make MSC good candidates for applications in tissue regeneration.

MSC are among the most highly studied types of adult stem cells. They include cells derived from nearly all tissues comprising the human body. Initially, these cells were considered to have a limited regenerative capacity, restricted to giving rise only to components of their tissue of origin. However, it is now apparent that as well as maintaining host tissue homeostasis, they can, under specific conditions, differentiate into phenotypes other than their tissue or tissues of origin.[21,27] Although MSC have limited differentiation capacity compared with embryonic stem cells, they are easily accessible and immunocompatible and are associated with fewer ethical concerns, making them very good candidates for regenerative medicine applications. Specifically, MSC of dental origin have become an attractive target for use in periodontal regeneration.

DEFINING PROPERTIES OF MESENCHYMAL STEM CELLS

MSC have several defining features that have been well documented. Specifically, these features include (i) their capacity to differentiate, under appropriate culture conditions, into at least 3 distinct lineages, such as osteoblasts, chondrocytes, and adipocytes; (ii) positive expression of cell surface markers, such as CD73, CD90, CD105, and CD166; (iii) an ability of individual clonal populations to regenerate the stromal microenvironment of their tissue of origin, when implanted into immunocompromised mice; and (4) ability for self-renewal following serial transplantations in vivo.[28,29] Another important criterion for defining the function and potency of different MSC-like populations is the assessment of their production of cytokines and growth factors associated with stem cell survival, angiogenesis, and immune cell responses.[30]

Given the complexities and distinctiveness of various stem cell populations, the above fundamental phenotypic and functional features of different MSC populations must be recognized. When studying MSC, the above-described features should be recognized as a minimum set of standards for studying their biology. This minimum set of standards will become increasingly important as studies move from in vitro and animal studies into clinical applications for humans using these unique and highly versatile cells.

CELLS WITH POTENTIAL FOR USE IN PERIODONTAL REGENERATION

Stem cells from both extraoral and intraoral sources have been studied for their potential to be used in periodontal regeneration applications. To date, most studies have investigated MSC derived from a variety of tissue sources in preclinical animal studies for the treatment and regeneration of the periodontium. With ever-increasing evidence that this is a viable technology, reports of human clinical trials are now beginning to appear in the literature.

Multipotent stem cells that can differentiate into tissue-specific cells have been isolated and characterized from all dental tissues (except enamel).[31] Indeed, for some time, the regenerative capacity of the periodontium has been recognized, and this has been attributed to the presence of residual multipotent progenitor cells responsible for the development of the periodontium.[32–36] Importantly, dental tissue–derived MSC tend to be relatively committed in their regenerative potency because of the fact that dental tissues do not undergo continuous remodeling, as do other tissues with higher turnover such as bone.[37]

Dental pulp stem cells (DPSC) were the first dental MSC to be isolated and characterized.[38] Following their discovery, MSCs were identified in exfoliated deciduous teeth (SHED), periodontal ligament stem cells (PDLSC), the stem cells from apical papilla (SCAP), the dental follicle, and gingiva.[39–44] Each of these MSC populations varies with regards to their growth and differentiation capacities and general gene and protein expression profiles. Whether these differences relate specifically to their specific niche origins remains to be established. Given their specialized sites of origin, these intraoral dental stem cells have been studied for their potential to be used in tissue engineering-based cell therapies for periodontal regeneration in both animals and humans (**Fig. 1**).

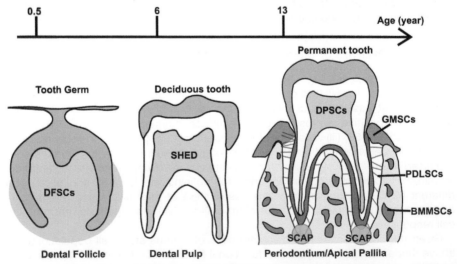

Fig. 1. Intraoral sources of MSC. Developing teeth: apical papilla; dental follicle. Children: exfoliated primary tooth pulp. Adult: pulp; periodontal ligament; gingiva.

STEM CELLS OF DENTAL ORIGIN FOR PERIODONTAL REGENERATION
Periodontal Ligament Stem Cells

The identification and isolation of PDLSC from the periodontal ligament have made these cells obvious candidates for periodontal regeneration studies. These cells are critical for the maintenance of tissue homeostasis and have considerable regenerative capacity, being able to differentiate into many different cell types, including cemento-blasts, osteoblasts, adipocytes, and fibroblasts as well as cementum/ periodontal ligament (PDL)-like structures.[42,45,46]

There have been many studies conducted investigating the use of PDLSC for periodontal regeneration. One systematic review concluded that irrespective of the defect type and animal model used, PDLSC implantation can be expected to result in a beneficial outcome for periodontal regeneration.[47] Furthermore, it was concluded that there was sufficient evidence from preclinical animal studies to warrant progression to human studies.[47] Accordingly, human trials using PDLSC for periodontal regeneration have commenced. Two recent reviews have been published assessing the outcomes of these studies.[48,49] The evidence to date indicates that although these cells are safe to use, the impact on periodontal regeneration is limited with some improvements noted, but also large heterogeneity was noted most likely because of variations in sample size and study protocols. Until large-scale, high-quality randomized clinical trials can be carried out, evidence to support the use of these cells for periodontal regeneration remains equivocal.

Dental Pulp Stem Cells

DPSC were the first dental stem cells to be identified.[38] Given that dental pulp is similar to bone marrow, being a highly vascularized tissue, it is not surprising that MSC have been found in this tissue. DPSC can form mineralized tissues and have the capacity for colony formation and high proliferation rates in vitro and expression of cell surface markers similar to those found on endothelial cells, smooth muscle cells, osteoblasts, and fibroblasts.[38] More recently, it has been determined that DPSC have higher proliferation rates, a lower rate of senescence, and enhanced osteogenic capacity compared with nondental MSC in vitro.[50] These cells demonstrated good periodontal regenerative capacity in a porcine periodontitis model. DPSC show superior resistance to subculture and inflammation-induced senescence and could be suitable for tissue engineering within an inflammatory environment. The utility of DPSC for periodontal regeneration is now well documented. Nevertheless, a recent systematic review concluded that periodontal regeneration, although DPSC could facilitate periodontal regeneration, was not as effective as PDLSC.[51]

STEM CELLS FROM HUMAN EXFOLIATED DECIDUOUS TEETH

Stem cells have been derived from the residual pulp of human exfoliated deciduous teeth.[41] Despite being of dental pulp origin, SHED are unique and distinct from adult DPSC in terms of their appearance, clonal and colony formation capacity, in vivo bone formation, and inability to form dentin-pulp-like tissue.[41] Interestingly, SHED have higher proliferation rates and higher expression of genes involved in producing cytokines responsible for cell proliferation and extracellular matrix synthesis.[52] To date, no studies have been reported on the use of SHED for periodontal regeneration.

Stem Cells from Apical Papilla

MSC have been isolated from the apical papilla, a complex organ comprising a collection of cells involved in the development of the tooth root and dental pulp. The cells have been termed SCAP.[43] Because of their association with tooth root development, these cells appear to have better regenerative capacity than other stem cells of dental origin.[43,44] SCAP can form odontoblast-like cells and adipocytes in vitro and also express several neurologic cell markers.[43,44,53] A good source of SCAP is from extracted third molars with incomplete root formation.

SCAP have the potential for use in the regeneration of the dentin/pulp complex and bioroot engineering.[43,44] An early study demonstrated that SCAP together with PDLSC in a prefabricated hydroxyapatite/tricalcium phosphate (HA/TCP) scaffold carrier regenerated a functional root/periodontal complex that could support a porcelain crown in miniature pigs.[43] More recently, a study has demonstrated that in a porcine model, local injection of SCAP into periodontal defects resulted in periodontal regeneration, indicating that these cells could be a useful source of dental-derived stem cells for periodontal regeneration.[54] No human studies have been carried out to date.

Dental Follicle Stem Cells

The dental follicle is a critical structural component of tooth development and is also a good source of MSC termed dental follicle stem cells (DFSC).[39] DFSC can be sourced from unerupted or impacted third molars. Although some studies have demonstrated the capacity of these cells to regenerate bone when implanted subcutaneously or into bony defects, there are no studies to date investigating the use of DFSC in periodontal regeneration of human periodontal defects.[55-57]

Gingival Mesenchymal Stem Cells

Although the multipotent potential of gingival fibroblasts has been recognized for a long time,[45] it is not until recently that mesenchymal stem cells from gingival tissues have been studied.[58-60] These cells demonstrate high proliferation rates, a stable morphology, and osteogenic capacity in vitro.[58,60-62] Gingival mesenchymal stem cells (GMSC) can promote bone formation in vivo when implanted into calvarial critical-size defects and periodontal defects in animals.[63,64] GMSC appear to have properties that are very similar to PDLSC.[65] GMSC have been studied for their capacity to assist in periodontal regeneration in several animal models (pig and dog). These studies have demonstrated that GMSC possess good periodontal regenerative potential, facilitating newly formed bone, cementum, and periodontal ligament fibers.[66,67] Although these cells have been proposed to be a good source of MSC-like cells for periodontal regeneration because of their easy availability and robust in vitro characteristics,[59] no human studies using these cells for periodontal regeneration have been carried out to date.

EXTRAORAL STEM CELLS FOR PERIODONTAL REGENERATION
Bone Marrow–Derived Mesenchymal Stem Cells

There are 3 major stem cell populations residing within the bone marrow: hematopoietic stem cells, angioblasts, and bone marrow stromal stem cells (BMSSC).[21,68-70]

These cells have considerable capacity to proliferate and expand in vitro and can differentiate into multiple cell lineages.[22,71,72] Accordingly, they have been studied extensively for their regenerative capacity in a wide variety of tissues and diseases.[73] BMSSC have been used for transplantation into periodontal defects in animal models[74] and have been shown to have good potential to differentiate into cementoblasts, periodontal ligament fibroblasts, and alveolar bone osteoblasts in vivo.[75] Human trials using these cells for periodontal regeneration have been carried out. An early study demonstrated good clinical results when autologous, expanded bone marrow-derived MSC mixed with atelocollagen were transplanted into periodontal osseous defects at the time of periodontal surgery.[76] The results showed a 4-mm reduction in probing depths and reduction in intrabony defect depth as well as resolution of bleeding and interdental papilla regeneration.[76]

A recent systematic review has indicated that BMSSC do support periodontal regeneration, but the evidence to date is still low quality, and further larger studies are needed to confirm their clinical utility.[48]

Adipose Tissue Stem Cells

Adipose tissue is emerging as an excellent source of easily accessible multipotent MSC with properties very similar to BMSSC.[77] Emerging studies are now suggesting that ASC may be superior to BMSCC for use in regenerative medicine because they are easier to harvest, demonstrate less senescence in vitro, and produce a vast array of growth and immunomodulatory factors conducive for tissue regeneration.[78–80]

The osteogenic capacity of adipose stem cells has been studied in considerable detail and has led to the suggestion that these cells are among the most promising for use in cell-based bone regeneration.[81] The osteogenic effect may arise due to their ability to differentiate into osteoblasts as well as through paracrine mechanisms, facilitating the migration and differentiation of other precursor osteoprogenitors.[82,83]

Adipose tissue stem cells (ASC) have been studied for periodontal regeneration. An early study demonstrated that, in a mouse model, ASC could promote regeneration of a periodontal ligament-like structure along with the alveolar bone.[84]

A recent systematic review assessed 15 publications reporting on the in vivo use of adipose tissue/cell for periodontal regeneration. These preclinical studies reported a general improvement of bone and periodontal healing when adipose tissue cells were delivered in a variety of carrier vehicles. It was concluded that adipose-derived cells might contribute to bone and periodontal regeneration; however, no meta-analyses could be carried out because of the heterogeneity of the studies.[85] There is an ongoing need for more definitive, well-controlled, and large-scale studies before any definitive conclusions can be made. To date, no human clinical trials for periodontal regeneration using ASC have been reported.

Induced Pluripotent Stem Cells

Reprogramming adult somatic cells into a pluripotent stem cell state has been a landmark development in stem cell biology and regenerative medicine.[16–18] These cells are termed IPSC. Using this technology, large populations of adult-derived stem cells can be generated without the ethical concerns of using embryonic stem cells (**Fig. 2**). IPSC can be generated from cells obtained from any tissue, and because of their unlimited

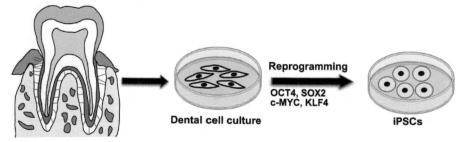

Fig. 2. IPSC cell production. Dental cells are cultured and "reprogrammed" by inserting several genes that instruct the cells to revert to an embryonic cell phenotype known as IPSCs.

growth capacity, that can provide an everlasting supply of stem cells. Although there has been considerable interest in using these cells in regenerative medicine, some features, such as potential for tumorigenicity and instability, significantly diminish their clinical utility.

IPSC have been generated from several dental-derived cells, including gingival, pulp, and periodontal ligament.[86–89] IPSC have been studied for their potential use in periodontal regeneration.[90,91] When implanted into periodontal defects, IPSC can significantly enhance regeneration and newly formed mineralized tissue formation. Interestingly, IPSC have been found to have the capacity to control acute and chronic inflammatory responses associated with the destruction of periodontal tissue when injected locally or systemically.[92]

CELL SHEETS FOR PERIODONTAL REGENERATION

Rather than using suspensions of cells embedded with various carrier scaffolds, the use of "cell sheets" has emerged as a novel alternative approach for periodontal tissue engineering (**Fig. 3**).[93,94] This technology uses temperature-responsive cell culture dishes modified to facilitate the removal of multilayered cell sheets. At normal culture conditions, the culture plate substrate is in a solid format, but it becomes more fluid when cooled and permits easy removal of the cell sheet from the culture plate.[95] This eliminates the need for enzymes to release the cells from the culture plate and is thus a noninvasive gentle process that maintains an intact extracellular matrix necessary for the viability of the cells at the time of transplantation.[96] Using this technology, the implanted cells presented to the defect site are less disrupted, allowing for critical cell-cell functions to continue operating. Several preclinical trials in animal models have demonstrated good periodontal regenerative outcomes with bone, periodontal ligament, and cementum confirmed histologically to have regenerated.[93,97] Transplants of cell sheets containing allogeneic cells in miniature swine have also demonstrated good periodontal tissue regenerative with no evidence of any adverse effects.[98] A recent study demonstrated favorable periodontal regeneration following the use of BMMSC cell sheets combined with multiphasic scaffolds in an ovine periodontal defect model.[99]

HUMAN CLINICAL TRIALS FOR CELL-BASED PERIODONTAL REGENERATION

With the demonstration that MSC can result in safe and efficacious periodontal regeneration in animal models, the time has come for the field to move on to human clinical trials.[47] Early case reports on the use of autologous periodontal cells and other MSC began to appear in the literature around 2005 (**Table 1**). An early single-arm and single-institute clinical study that commenced in 2011 investigated the potential use of autologous PDLSC sheets for periodontal regeneration. They reported that the therapeutic effects were sustained over 4.5 years with no serious side effects.[100] The first

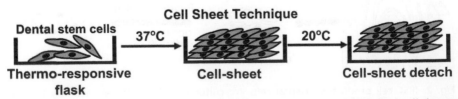

Cell Sheet Technique

Dental stem cells   37°C   **Cell-sheet**   20°C   **Cell-sheet detach**

Thermo-responsive flask

Fig. 3. Cell sheet production. Dental cells are cultured to produce multilayered cell sheets.

Table 1
Use of autologous periodontal cells and other mesenchymal stem cells for periodontal regeneration

Reference	Study Format	Stem Cell Type	Number of Defects/Subjects	Carrier Vehicle	Defect	Outcome	Complications/Safety Issues
Akbay et al,[111] 2005	Randomized clinical trial	Periodontal ligament graft Autologous	20/10 No controls	PDL scraped from tooth root; no carrier used	Mandibular class II furcation	Improved CAL, pocket, bone fill Increased gingival recession	No foreign body response noted
Yamada et al,[76] 2006	Case report	Bone marrow stromal stem cells Autologous	1/1	Platelet-rich plasma	Intrabony	Improved CAL, pocket depth, bone fill	Not assessed
Feng et al,[112] 2010	Pilot study/case report	Periodontal ligament stem cells Autologous	16/3	Hydroxyapatite/tricalcium phosphate	Intrabony	Improved CAL, pocket depth Increased gingival recession	Nil
McAlliser,[113] 2011	Case report	Bone marrow stromal stem cells Allogeneic	2/2	Commercial cellular allograft bone matrix (Osteocel; ACE Surgical Supply)	1 × intrabony 1 × grade II furcation	Improved pocket depth, bone fill	Not assessed
Koo et al,[114] 2012	Case report	Bone marrow stromal stem cells Allogeneic	1/1	Osteocel; NuVasive, San Diego, CA, USA covered with a resorbable membrane (DynaMatrix; Keystone Dental, Burlington, MA, USA)	Intrabony	Improved CAL, pocket depth	Not assessed

(continued on next page)

Table 1
(continued)

Reference	Study Format	Stem Cell Type	Number of Defects/ Subjects	Carrier Vehicle	Defect	Outcome	Complications/ Safety Issues
Yamada et al,[115] 2013	Case series	Bone marrow stromal stem cells Autologous	17/17	Platelet-rich plasma	Intrabony	Improved CAL, pocket depth	Nil
Rosen,[116] 2013	Case report	Bone marrow stromal stem cells Allogeneic	1/1	Osteocel; NuVasive, covered with an amnion-chorion membrane (BioXclude; Snoasis Medical, Denver, CO, USA)	Mandibular grade III furcation	Improved pocket depth Increased gingival recession	Not assessed
Aimetti et al,[117] 2014	Case report	Dental pulp Autologous	1/1	Dental pulp cell suspension from dissociated third molar pulp mixed into collagen sponge	Intrabony	Improved pocket depth, CAL, bone fill	Not assessed
Aimetti et al,[118] 2015	Case series	Dental pulp Autologous	4/4	Dental pulp cell suspension from dissociated third molar pulp mixed into collagen sponge	Intrabony	Improved CAL, pocket depth, bone fill	Not assessed
Baba et al,[119] 2016	Phase I/II clinical trial	Bone marrow stromal stem cell Autologous	10/10 No treatment controls	Platelet-rich plasma	Intrabony	Improved CAL, pocket depth, bone fill	Nil
Li et al,[120] 2016	Case report	Inflamed dental pulp stem cells Autologous	2/2	β-Tricalcium phosphate	Intrabony	Improved pocket depth	Nil

Study	Study type	Cell source	Sample	Scaffold/material	Defect	Outcomes	Adverse events
Chen et al,[121] 2016	Randomized clinical trial	Periodontal ligament stem cells Autologous	41/30 Test = 21 Control = 20 Bio-Oss with GTR membrane (no cells)	Bovine-derived bone mineral materials (Bio-Oss)	Intrabony	Improved CAL, pocket depth, bone fill No difference with the control group	Nil
KI et al,[122] 2017	Case report	Periodontal ligament and cementum scraping Autogenous	1/1	Gelatin sponge (Abgel)	Intrabony	Improved CAL, pocket depth	Not assessed
Aimetti et al,[123] 2018	Case series	Dental pulp Allogeneic	11/11	Dental pulp cell suspension from dissociated third-molar pulp mixed into collagen sponge	Intrabony	Improved CAL, pocket depth, bone fill	Not assessed
Ferraroti et al,[124] 2018	Randomized clinical trial	Dental pulp stem cells Autologous	29/29 Test = 15 Control = 14 (collagen sponge without cells)	Collagen sponge (Condress; Istituto Gentili, Milano, Italy)	Intrabony	Improved CAL, pocket depth, bone fill, increased gingival recession	Not assessed
Hernandez-Monjaraz et al,[125] 2018	Case report Allogeneic	Deciduous tooth pulp Allogeneic	1/1	Lyophilized Collagen-polyvinylpyrrolidone sponge	Intrabony	Improved pocket depth, bone fill	Nil

(continued on next page)

Table 1
(continued)

Reference	Study Format	Stem Cell Type	Number of Defects/ Subjects	Carrier Vehicle	Defect	Outcome	Complications/ Safety Issues
Iwata et al,[100] 2018	Single-arm and single-institute clinical study	Autogenous periodontal cell sheets	10/10 No controls	Cell sheets laid adjacent to root surface and defect filled with β-tricalcium phosphate	Intrabony	Improved CAL, probing depth, bone fill	Nil
Shalini & Vandana,[126] 2018	Randomized clinical trial	Autologous periodontal ligament cells	28 subjects: 14 control 14 test	PDL scraped from tooth root	Infrabony	Improved CAL, probing depth, bone fill, bone density	Not assessed
Hernandez-Monjaraz et al,[127] 2020	Case/control clinical study	Deciduous tooth pulp Allogeneic	22/22 Test = 11 Control = 11 (carrier with no cells)	Lyophilized polyvinylpyrrolidone Sponge			Nil

human clinical trials using BMSSC and PDLSC were reported in 2016. To date, cells from a variety of sources, including bone marrow, dental pulp, and periodontal ligament, have been studied with mixed results.[48] A systematic review of these studies concluded that there is only low-quality evidence demonstrating that MSC use for periodontal regeneration results in generally small gains. Because of the heterogeneity of the studies and low sample sizes, conclusions are difficult to make, and more definitive studies are needed.[48]

FUTURE CELL-BASED THERAPIES FOR PERIODONTAL REGENERATION
Allogeneic Cell Sources and Establishment of Cell Banks

Autologous transplantation of cells has been shown to be both safe and efficacious (see **Table 1**). However, difficulties can be encountered with the use of autologous cells, particularly from dental sources. If there are no redundant or suitable teeth for extraction, then the primary source of dental-derived stem cells becomes nonexistent. Notwithstanding this issue, other problems, such as the generation of standardized and stable autologous cell populations and the length of time it takes to produce sufficient cells from the primary source, all lead to substantial logistic difficulties in the use of autologous cells. Therefore, allogeneic cells have been proposed as an alternative source of cells for periodontal tissue engineering and regeneration.[101] In this context, dental-derived stem cells can be generated in vitro using strict production protocols to produce standardized populations of cells for future use. Extracted teeth, such as third molars, could serve as an ideal source of such cells. Accordingly, the concept of tissue banking of human dental-derived stem cells has been proposed.[102] Although this is an attractive concept, issues such as the risk of infection from donor cells remain a concern and require stringent safety and efficacy protocols to be developed. In general autologous cells are tolerated very well and do not display significant adverse graft/host reactions.

Embryonic Stem/Induced Pluripotent Cells

In the context of cell banking, IPSCs offer considerable potential. As detailed earlier, IPSC are unique stem cell populations generated in vitro through genetic manipulation and reprogramming of somatic cells into cells with an embryonic stem cell phenotype regarding morphology, gene expression profiles, proliferation, and differentiation capacities, but without ethical concerns of embryonic stem cells.[16–18] Therefore, the potential for these cells to be propagated in vitro and stored in a tissue bank for future use is an attractive idea. Several reports detailing the production of IPSC from dental-derived adult cells are sourced from gingival, pulp, and periodontal ligament tissues.[86–88] Early preclinical studies have demonstrated the potential of these cells to be used for periodontal regeneration. IPSC have been studied for their potential use in periodontal regeneration.[90,91] However, to date, no human trials have been reported because of ongoing concerns regarding the safety and efficacy of these cells.

Conditioned Medium of Cultured Mesenchymal Stem Cells

One way stem cells exert their regenerative capacity is through the secretion of cytokines, growth factors, and other bioactive proteins that can drive tissue regeneration. It has been suggested that the conditioned media produced by these cells in culture may have regenerative instructive messages that could be used for tissue regeneration. The use of a conditioned medium may overcome limitations of low survival rates and the potential tumorigenicity associated with cell transplantation.

Proof-of-concept studies have been reported in preclinical animal periodontal defect models using conditioned medium from cultured bone marrow MSC, PDLSC, and gingival stem cells.[103–106] These studies have confirmed that these cells produce, in vitro, bioactive proteins, such as extracellular matrix proteins, enzymes, angiogenic factors, insulin-like growth factor-1, vascular endothelial growth factor, transforming growth factor-beta 1, and hepatocyte growth factor. These factors have been attributed to the significantly greater alveolar bone, and cementum regeneration is noted when applied into periodontal defects. To date, no human studies using conditioned medium have been published.

Exosomes

Another component of the MSC secretome is the release of extracellular vesicles called exosomes. Exosomes are membrane-bound extracellular vesicles that are produced in the endosomal compartment of eukaryotic cells and are released from cells upon fusion with the plasma membrane. Like conditioned medium, extracellular vesicles attract considerable interest as potential agents to be harnessed for cell-based periodontal regeneration. There are few ethical impediments to using extracellular vesicles (and cultured medium), and this technology accesses their easy acquisition and preservation and their amenity to long-term storage, sterilization, and packaging. There are 3 types of extracellular vesicles: (1) exosomes that arise via endocytosis, (2) microvesicles that are formed through budding of the cell membrane, and (3) apoptotic bodies that arise from programmed cell death. Interest in extracellular vesicles has arisen because of their involvement in various biological processes, including cell-cell communication, protein, nucleic acid transport, and cell metabolism. They can engage with cell surface proteins activating intercellular signaling pathways and can be involved in the activation of MSC tissue regeneration. Extracellular vesicle membrane proteins may interact with the cell surface and activate intercellular signaling pathways within progenitors and stem cells. EVs derived from stem/progenitor cells have the potential to mediate the regenerative responses of MSC.[107] Accordingly, EVs have attracted interest for their potential use in periodontal treatment and regeneration.[108–110] No human studies have been reported to date.

LIMITATIONS OF STEM CELL THERAPY FOR PERIODONTAL REGENERATION

Notwithstanding the overall potential use of MSC for periodontal regeneration, several issues still need to be addressed before this type of therapy can become mainstream clinical practice.

Further fundamental studies are needed using sufficient quantities of cells required for various clinical applications. Little is known about the biological regulatory processes necessary for stem cell differentiation and maturation into tissue-specific phenotypes. Another as yet poorly researched area is the study of controlling mechanisms for the regulation and prevention of transformation of MSC into cells with unwanted or carcinogenic potential. Finally, exploration of how the regenerative process can be controlled spatially and temporally is still poorly understood.

Another significant issue in using stem cell therapies is the cost of producing cells in large quantities required for in vivo implantation. Irrespective of whether autologous or allogeneic sources are used, the process of isolating, culturing, screening, and characterizing against specific stem cell checklists cannot be underestimated. These processes are still time-consuming and expensive, and this cost must ultimately be passed on to the end-user (the patient). Thus, to justify the cost, one will need to be very sure that the clinical benefit in terms of tissue regeneration, improvement of function, and longevity of the benefit is better than current gold-standard regenerative procedures. In addition to this, but also in line with the cost of production, is the development of strict good manufacturing procedures for the production of stem cells for periodontal regeneration. This will involve adherence to specific protocols to confirm the "stemness" of the cells in use[29] and specifications for purpose-built production facilities and safety protocols.

SUMMARY

Cell-based tissue engineering is an attractive prospect for periodontal regeneration. Many cells of both dental and nondental origin have been studied for their potential use in periodontal regeneration. New frontiers using cell-based products rather than whole cells are also gaining attention. To date, the clinical results using stem cell–based approaches for periodontal regeneration have been equivocal because of largely limited large-scale controlled clinical studies being carried out. There is no doubt that cell-based tissue engineering is a new and exciting field for periodontics. However, there is still a great deal of work needed before this technology can be used for clinical periodontal regenerative therapies. The field of regenerative periodontics is very complex, and in order for it to become a mainstream clinical reality, scientists and clinicians will need to unite their resources. Scientific input will be needed from many differing but interrelated fields. For example, input from diverse fields, such as immunology, cell biology, molecular biology, nanotechnology, materials science, and microbiology, to name a few, will be needed to address issues, such as (i) understanding host reactions to the implanted cells and also ensuring immunologic safety; (ii) production of cell-based products with the required biologic functionality; (iii) construction of implantable biologic materials with all of the necessary instructional messages to produce clinically predictable periodontal regeneration; (iv) safe and contaminant-free surgical delivery into the recipient site; and (v) maintaining the regenerated tissues in a fully functional state. Of course, the final hurdle to overcome will be to demonstrate cost/benefit efficacy and proof that cell-based periodontal regenerative procedures can enhance the longevity and survival rate of the treated teeth.

CLINICS CARE POINTS

- Currently, periodontal regeneration is recognized as being biologically possible but clinically unpredictable and remains an elusive goal.
- Until large scale high quality randomized clinical trials can be carried out evidence to support the use of stem cells for periodontal regeneration remains equivocal.
- There is no doubt that the field of cell-based tissue engineering is a new and exciting field for periodontics. However there is still a great deal of work needed before this technology can be utilised for clinical periodontal regenerative therapies.

ACKNOWLEDGMENTS

The authors thank Pingping Han for assistance with the preparation of the figures.

DISCLOSURE

Both authors declare they have no commercial or financial conflicts of interest. Any original research of the authors referred to in this review was funded by the National Health and Medical Research Council of Australia.

REFERENCES

1. Murakami S, Bartold M, Meyle J, et al. Group c. consensus paper. Periodontal regeneration–fact or fiction? J Int Acad Periodontol 2015;17(1 Suppl):54–6.
2. Aimetti M, Citterio F, Cairo F. Pocket resolution in regenerative treatment of intrabony defects with papilla preservation techniques: a systematic review and meta-analysis of randomized clinical trials. J Clin Periodontol 2021;48(6): 843–58.
3. Needleman IG, Worthington HV, Giedrys-Leeper E, et al. Guided tissue regeneration for periodontal infra-bony defects. Cochrane Database Syst Rev 2006;(2):CD001724.
4. Nibali L. Guest editorial: time to reflect on new evidence about periodontal regenerative surgery of intrabony defects. J Clin Periodontol 2021;48(4):557–9.
5. Bartold P, McCulloch C, Naryanan A, et al. Tissue engineering: a new paradigm for periodontal regeneration based on cell and molecular biology. Periodontol 2000 2000;24:253–69.
6. Becker W, Becker BE. Periodontal regeneration: a contemporary re-evaluation. Periodontol 2000 1999;19:104–14.
7. Bordin S, Narayanan AS, Reddy J, et al. Fibroblast subtypes in the periodontium. A possible role in connective tissue regeneration and periodontal reattachment. J Periodont Res 1984;19:642–4.
8. Bordin S, Page R, Narayanan A. Heterogeneity of normal diploid fibroblasts: isolation and characterisation of one phenotype. Science 1984;223:171–3.
9. Ivanovski S, Haase HR, Bartold PM. Expression of bone matrix protein mRNAs by primary and cloned cultures of the regenerative phenotype of human periodontal fibroblasts. J Dent Res 2001;80(7):1665–71.
10. Ivanovski S, Haase HR, Bartold PM. Isolation and characterization of fibroblasts derived from regenerating human periodontal defects. Arch Oral Biol 2001; 46(8):679–88.
11. Smith A. A glossary for stem-cell biology. Nature 2006;441(7097):1060.
12. Morrison SJ, Shah NM, Anderson DJ. Regulatory mechanisms in stem cell biology. Cell 1997;88(3):287–98.
13. Martin GR. Isolation of a pluripotent cell line from early mouse embryos cultured in medium conditioned by teratocarcinoma stem cells. Proc Natl Acad Sci U S A 1981;78(12):7634–8.
14. Thomson JA, Itskovitz-Eldor J, Shapiro SS, et al. Embryonic stem cell lines derived from human blastocysts. Science 1998;282(5391):1145–7.
15. Evans MJ, Kaufman MH. Establishment in culture of pluripotent cells from mouse embryos. Nature 1981;292(5819):154–6.
16. Takahashi K, Yamanaka S. Induction of pluripotent stem cells from mouse embryonic and adult fibroblast cultures by defined factors. Cell 2006;126(4): 663–76.
17. Takahashi K, Tanabe K, Ohnuki M, et al. Induction of pluripotent stem cells from adult human fibroblasts by defined factors. Cell 2007;131(5):861–72.
18. Yu J, Vodyanik MA, Smuga-Otto K, et al. Induced pluripotent stem cell lines derived from human somatic cells. Science 2007;318(5858):1917–20.
19. Bongso A, Fong C-Y, Gauthaman K. Taking stem cells to the clinic: major challenges. J Cell Biochem 2008;105(6):1352–60.
20. Lee H, Park J, Forget BG, et al. Induced pluripotent stem cells in regenerative medicine: an argument for continued research on human embryonic stem cells. Regen Med 2009;4(5):759–69.

21. Pittenger MF, Mackay AM, Beck SC, et al. Multilineage potential of adult human mesenchymal stem cells. Science 1999;284(5411):143–7.
22. Gronthos S, Zannettino ACW, Hay SJ, et al. Molecular and cellular characterisation of highly purified stromal stem cells derived from human bone marrow. J Cell Sci 2003;116(Pt 9):1827–35.
23. Horwitz EM, Prockop DJ, Fitzpatrick LA, et al. Transplantability and therapeutic effects of bone marrow-derived mesenchymal cells in children with osteogenesis imperfecta. Nat Med 1999;5(3):309–13.
24. Jiang YH, Jahagirdar BN, Reinhardt RL, et al. Pluripotency of mesenchymal stem cells derived from adult marrow. Nature 2002;418(6893):41–9.
25. Pereira RF, Halford KW, Ohara MD, et al. Cultured adherent cells from marrow can serve as long lasting precursor cells for bone, cartilage, and lung in irradiated mice. Proc Natl Acad Sci U S A 1995;92(11):4857–61.
26. Smith JR, Pochampally R, Perry A, et al. Isolation of a highly clonogenic and multipotential subfraction of adult stem cells from bone marrow stroma. Stem Cells 2004;22(5):823–31.
27. Bianco P, Robey PG. Stem cells in tissue engineering. Nature 2001;414(6859): 118–21.
28. Dominici M, Le Blanc K, Mueller I, et al. Minimal criteria for defining multipotent mesenchymal stromal cells. The International Society for Cellular Therapy position statement. Cytotherapy 2006;8(4):315–7.
29. Bartold PM, Gronthos S. Standardization of criteria defining periodontal ligament stem cells. J Dent Res 2017;96(5):487–90.
30. Konala VBR, Mamidi MK, Bhonde R, et al. The current landscape of the mesenchymal stromal cell secretome: a new paradigm for cell-free regeneration. Cytotherapy 2016;18(1):13–24.
31. Chen FM, Sun HH, Lu H, et al. Stem cell-delivery therapeutics for periodontal tissue regeneration. Biomaterials 2012;33(27):6320–44.
32. Beertsen W, McCulloch CAG, Sodek J. The periodontal ligament: a unique, multifunctional connective tissue. Periodontol 2000 1997;13:20–40.
33. Boyko GA, Melcher AH, Brunette DM. Formation of new periodontal ligament by periodontal ligament cells implanted in vivo after culture in vitro. A preliminary study of transplanted roots in the dog. J Periodontal Res 1981;16(1):73–88.
34. Gould TRL, Melcher AH, Brunette DM. Migration and division of progenitor cell populations in periodontal ligament after wounding. J Periodontal Res 1980; 15(1):20–42.
35. Liu HW, Yacobi R, Savion N, et al. A collagenous cementum-derived attachment protein is a marker for progenitors of the mineralized tissue-forming cell lineage of the periodontal ligament. J Bone Miner Res 1997;12(10):1691–9.
36. Ivanovski S, Gronthos S, Shi S, et al. Stem cells in the periodontal ligament. Oral Dis 2006;12(4):358–63.
37. Huang GT, Gronthos S, Shi S. Mesenchymal stem cells derived from dental tissues vs. those from other sources: their biology and role in regenerative medicine. J Dent Res 2009;88(9):792–806.
38. Gronthos S, Mankani M, Brahim J, et al. Postnatal human dental pulp stem cells (DPSCs) in vitro and in vivo. Proc Natl Acad Sci U S A 2000;97(25):13625–30.
39. Morsczeck C, Gotz W, Schierholz J, et al. Isolation of precursor cells (PCs) from human dental follicle of wisdom teeth. Matrix Biol 2005;24(2):155–65.
40. Zhang QZ, Nguyen AL, Yu WH, et al. Human oral mucosa and gingiva: a unique reservoir for mesenchymal stem cells. J Dent Res 2012;91(11):1011–8.

41. Miura M, Gronthos S, Zhao MR, et al. SHED: stem cells from human exfoliated deciduous teeth. Proc Natl Acad Sci U S A 2003;100(10):5807–12.

42. Seo BM, Miura M, Gronthos S, et al. Investigation of multipotent postnatal stem cells from human periodontal ligament. Lancet 2004;364(9429):149–55.

43. Sonoyama W, Liu Y, Fang D, et al. Mesenchymal stem cell-mediated functional tooth regeneration in swine. PLoS One 2006;1:e79.

44. Sonoyama W, Liu Y, Yamaza T, et al. Characterization of the apical papilla and its residing stem cells from human immature permanent teeth: a pilot study. J Endod 2008;34(2):166–71.

45. McCulloch CA, Bordin S. Role of fibroblast subpopulations in periodontal physiology and pathology. J Periodontal Res 1991;26(3 Pt 1):144–54.

46. Isaka J, Ohazama A, Kobayashi M, et al. Participation of periodontal ligament cells with regeneration of alveolar bone. J Periodontol 2001;72(3):314–23.

47. Bright R, Hynes K, Gronthos S, et al. Periodontal ligament-derived cells for periodontal regeneration in animal models: a systematic review. J Periodontal Res 2015;50(2):160–72.

48. Novello S, Debouche A, Philippe M, et al. Clinical application of mesenchymal stem cells in periodontal regeneration: a systematic review and meta-analysis. J Periodontal Res 2020;55(1):1–12.

49. Yamada Y, Nakamura-Yamada S, Konoki R, et al. Promising advances in clinical trials of dental tissue-derived cell-based regenerative medicine. Stem Cell Res Ther 2020;11(1):175.

50. Ma LS, Hu JC, Cao Y, et al. Maintained properties of aged dental pulp stem cells for superior periodontal tissue regeneration. Aging Dis 2019;10(4):793–806.

51. Amghar-Maach S, Gay-Escoda C, Sanchez-Garces MA. Regeneration of periodontal bone defects with dental pulp stem cells grafting: systematic review. J Clin Exp Dent 2019;11(4):e373–81.

52. Nakamura S, Yamada Y, Katagiri W, et al. Stem cell proliferation pathways comparison between human exfoliated deciduous teeth and dental pulp stem cells by gene expression profile from promising dental pulp. J Endod 2009;35(11):1536–42.

53. Abe S, Yamaguchi S, Amagasa T. Multilineage cells from apical pulp of human tooth with immature apex. Oral Sci Int 2007;45–58.

54. Li G, Han N, Zhang X, et al. Local injection of allogeneic stem cells from apical papilla enhanced periodontal tissue regeneration in minipig model of periodontitis. Biomed Res Int 2018;2018:3960798.

55. Tsuchiya S, Ohshima S, Yamakoshi Y, et al. Osteogenic differentiation capacity of porcine dental follicle progenitor cells. Connect Tissue Res 2010;51(3):197–207.

56. Park BW, Kang EJ, Byun JH, et al. In vitro and in vivo osteogenesis of human mesenchymal stem cells derived from skin, bone marrow and dental follicle tissues. Differentiation 2012;83(5):249–59.

57. Rezai-Rad M, Bova JF, Orooji M, et al. Evaluation of bone regeneration potential of dental follicle stem cells for treatment of craniofacial defects. Cytotherapy 2015;17(11):1572–81.

58. Fournier BP, Ferre FC, Couty L, et al. Multipotent progenitor cells in gingival connective tissue. Tissue Eng Part A 2010;16(9):2891–9.

59. Fawzy El-Sayed KM, Dorfer CE. Gingival mesenchymal stem/progenitor cells: a unique tissue engineering gem. Stem Cells Int 2016;2016:7154327.

60. El-Sayed KM, Paris S, Graetz C, et al. Isolation and characterisation of human gingival margin-derived STRO-1/MACS(+) and MACS(−) cell populations. Int J Oral Sci 2015;7(2):80–8.

61. Tomar GB, Srivastava RK, Gupta N, et al. Human gingiva-derived mesenchymal stem cells are superior to bone marrow-derived mesenchymal stem cells for cell therapy in regenerative medicine. Biochem Biophys Res Commun 2010;393(3): 377–83.

62. Mitrano TI, Grob MS, Carrion F, et al. Culture and characterization of mesenchymal stem cells from human gingival tissue. J Periodontol 2010;81(6):917–25.

63. Wang F, Yu M, Yan X, et al. Gingiva-derived mesenchymal stem cell-mediated therapeutic approach for bone tissue regeneration. Stem Cells Dev 2011; 20(12):2093–102.

64. Yu M, Ge S, Wang F, et al. The role of systemically delivered bone marrow-derived mesenchymal stem cells in the regeneration of periodontal tissues. Int J Oral Maxillofac Implants 2013;28(6):e503–11.

65. Santamaria S, Sanchez N, Sanz M, et al. Comparison of periodontal ligament and gingiva-derived mesenchymal stem cells for regenerative therapies. Clin Oral Investig 2017;21(4):1095–102.

66. Yu X, Ge S, Chen S, et al. Human gingiva-derived mesenchymal stromal cells contribute to periodontal regeneration in beagle dogs. Cells Tissues Organs 2013;198(6):428–37.

67. Fawzy El-Sayed KM, Mekhemar MK, Beck-Broichsitter BE, et al. Periodontal regeneration employing gingival margin-derived stem/progenitor cells in conjunction with il-1ra-hydrogel synthetic extracellular matrix. J Clin Periodontol 2015;42(5):448–57.

68. Friedenstein AJ, Chailakhjan RK, Lalykina KS. The development of fibroblast colonies in monolayer cultures of guinea-pig bone marrow and spleen cells. Cell Tissue Kinet 1970;3(4):393–403.

69. Gronthos S, Chen S, Wang CY, et al. Telomerase accelerates osteogenesis of bone marrow stromal stem cells by upregulation of cbfa1, osterix, and osteocalcin. J Bone Miner Res 2003;18(4):716–22.

70. Owen M, Friedenstein AJ. Stromal stem cells: marrow-derived osteogenic precursors. Ciba Found Symp 1988;136:42–60.

71. Kuznetsov SA, Krebsbach PH, Satomura K, et al. Single-colony derived strains of human marrow stromal fibroblasts form bone after transplantation in vivo. J Bone Miner Res 1997;12(9):1335–47.

72. Menicanin D, Bartold PM, Zannettino AC, et al. Identification of a common gene expression signature associated with immature clonal mesenchymal cell populations derived from bone marrow and dental tissues. Stem Cells Dev 2010; 19(10):1501–10.

73. Bianco P, Riminucci M, Gronthos S, et al. Bone marrow stromal stem cells: nature, biology, and potential applications. Stem Cells 2001;19(3):180–92.

74. Kawaguchi H, Hirachi A, Hasegawa N, et al. Enhancement of periodontal tissue regeneration by transplantation of bone marrow mesenchymal stem cells. J Periodontol 2004;75(9):1281–7.

75. Hasegawa N, Kawaguchi H, Hirachi A, et al. Behavior of transplanted bone marrow-derived mesenchymal stem cells in periodontal defects. J Periodontol 2006;77(6):1003–7.

76. Yamada Y, Ueda M, Hibi H, et al. A novel approach to periodontal tissue regeneration with mesenchymal stem cells and platelet-rich plasma using tissue

engineering technology: a clinical case report. Int J Periodontics Restorative Dent 2006;26(4):363–9.

77. Bacakova L, Zarubova J, Travnickova M, et al. Stem cells: their source, potency and use in regenerative therapies with focus on adipose-derived stem cells - a review. Biotechnol Adv 2018;36(4):1111–26.

78. Hsiao ST, Asgari A, Lokmic Z, et al. Comparative analysis of paracrine factor expression in human adult mesenchymal stem cells derived from bone marrow, adipose, and dermal tissue. Stem Cells Dev 2012;21(12):2189–203.

79. Ding DC, Chou HL, Hung WT, et al. Human adipose-derived stem cells cultured in keratinocyte serum free medium: donor's age does not affect the proliferation and differentiation capacities. J Biomed Sci 2013;20:59.

80. Varghese J, Griffin M, Mosahebi A, et al. Systematic review of patient factors affecting adipose stem cell viability and function: implications for regenerative therapy. Stem Cell Res Ther 2017;8(1):45.

81. Lindroos B, Suuronen R, Miettinen S. The potential of adipose stem cells in regenerative medicine. Stem Cell Rev 2011;7(2):269–91.

82. de Girolamo L, Sartori MF, Albisetti W, et al. Osteogenic differentiation of human adipose-derived stem cells: comparison of two different inductive media. J Tissue Eng Regen Med 2007;1(2):154–7.

83. Tajima S, Tobita M, Orbay H, et al. Direct and indirect effects of a combination of adipose-derived stem cells and platelet-rich plasma on bone regeneration. Tissue Eng Part A 2015;21(5–6):895–905.

84. Tobita M, Uysal AC, Ogawa R, et al. Periodontal tissue regeneration with adipose-derived stem cells. Tissue Eng Part A 2008;14(6):945–53.

85. Moreira Dziedzic DS, Mogharbel BF, Ferreira PE, et al. Transplantation of adipose-derived cells for periodontal regeneration: a systematic review. Curr Stem Cell Res Ther 2019;14(6):504–18.

86. Tamaoki N, Takahashi K, Tanaka T, et al. Dental pulp cells for induced pluripotent stem cell banking. J Dent Res 2010;89(8):773–8.

87. Wada N, Wang B, Lin NH, et al. Induced pluripotent stem cell lines derived from human gingival fibroblasts and periodontal ligament fibroblasts. J Periodontal Res 2011;46(4):438–47.

88. Nomura Y, Ishikawa M, Yashiro Y, et al. Human periodontal ligament fibroblasts are the optimal cell source for induced pluripotent stem cells. Histochem Cell Biol 2012;137(6):719–32.

89. Hynes K, Menichanin D, Bright R, et al. Induced pluripotent stem cells: a new frontier for stem cells in dentistry. J Dent Res 2015;94(11):1508–15.

90. Hynes K, Menicanin D, Han J, et al. Mesenchymal stem cells from IPSC cells facilitate periodontal regeneration. J Dent Res 2013;92(9):833–9.

91. Chien K-H, Chang Y-L, Wang M-L, et al. Promoting induced pluripotent stem cell-driven biomineralization and periodontal regeneration in rats with maxillary-molar defects using injectable bmp-6 hydrogel. Sci Rep 2018;8:114.

92. Hynes K, Bright R, Marino V, et al. Potential of iPSC-derived mesenchymal stromal cells for treating periodontal disease. Stem Cells Int 2018;2018:2601945.

93. Akizuki T, Oda S, Komaki M, et al. Application of periodontal ligament cell sheet for periodontal regeneration: a pilot study in beagle dogs. J Periodontal Res 2005;40(3):245–51.

94. Bartold PM, Gronthos S, Ivanovski S, et al. Tissue engineered periodontal products. J Periodontal Res 2016;51(1):1–15.

95. Hirose M, Kwon OH, Yamato M, et al. Creation of designed shape cell sheets that are noninvasively harvested and moved onto another surface. Biomacromolecules 2000;1(3):377–81.

96. Kushida A, Yamato M, Konno C, et al. Decrease in culture temperature releases monolayer endothelial cell sheets together with deposited fibronectin matrix from temperature-responsive culture surfaces. J Biomed Mater Res 1999; 45(4):355–62.

97. Tsumanuma Y, Iwata T, Washio K, et al. Comparison of different tissue-derived stem cell sheets for periodontal regeneration in a canine 1-wall defect model. Biomaterials 2011;32(25):5819–25.

98. Ding G, Liu Y, Wang W, et al. Allogeneic periodontal ligament stem cell therapy for periodontitis in swine. Stem Cells 2010;28(10):1829–38.

99. Vaquette C, Saifzadeh S, Farag A, et al. Periodontal tissue engineering with a multiphasic construct and cell sheets. J Dent Res 2019;98(6):673–81.

100. Iwata T, Yamato M, Washio K, et al. Periodontal regeneration with autologous periodontal ligament-derived cell sheets - a safety and efficacy study in ten patients. Regenerative Ther 2018;9:38–44.

101. Mrozik KM, Wada N, Marino V, et al. Regeneration of periodontal tissues using allogeneic periodontal ligament stem cells in an ovine model. Regen Med 2013; 8(6):711–23.

102. Vaithilingam RD, Safii SH, Baharuddin NA, et al. Establishing and managing a periodontal biobank for research: the sharing of experience. Oral Dis 2015; 21(1):E62–9.

103. Nagata M, Iwasaki K, Akazawa K, et al. Conditioned medium from periodontal ligament stem cells enhances periodontal regeneration. Tissue Eng Part A 2017;23(9–10):367–77.

104. Qiu JL, Wang XT, Zhou HW, et al. Enhancement of periodontal tissue regeneration by conditioned media from gingiva-derived or periodontal ligament-derived mesenchymal stem cells: a comparative study in rats. Stem Cell Res Ther 2020; 11(1):42.

105. Inukai T, Katagiri W, Yoshimi R, et al. Novel application of stem cell-derived factors for periodontal regeneration. Biochem Biophys Res Commun 2013;430(2): 763–8.

106. Kawai T, Katagiri W, Osugi M, et al. Secretomes from bone marrow-derived mesenchymal stromal cells enhance periodontal tissue regeneration. Cytotherapy 2015;17(4):369–81.

107. Yuan QL, Zhang YG, Chen Q. Mesenchymal stem cell (MSC)-derived extracellular vesicles: potential therapeutics as MSC trophic mediators in regenerative medicine. Anat Rec (Hoboken) 2020;303(6):1735–42.

108. Mohammed E, Khalil E, Sabry D. Effect of adipose-derived stem cells and their exo as adjunctive therapy to nonsurgical periodontal treatment: a histologic and histomorphometric study in rats. Biomolecules 2018;8(4):167.

109. Chew JRJ, Chuah SJ, Teo KYW, et al. Mesenchymal stem cell exosomes enhance periodontal ligament cell functions and promote periodontal regeneration. Acta Biomater 2019;89:252–64.

110. Novello S, Pellen-Mussi P, Jeanne S. Mesenchymal stem cell-derived small extracellular vesicles as cell-free therapy: perspectives in periodontal regeneration. J Periodontal Res 2021. https://doi.org/10.1111/jre.12866.

111. Akbay A, Baran C, Gunhan O, et al. Periodontal regenerative potential of autogenous periodontal ligament grafts in class ii furcation defects. J Periodontol 2005;76(4):595–604.

112. Feng F, Akiyama K, Liu Y, et al. Utility of PDL progenitors for in vivo tissue regeneration: a report of 3 cases. Oral Dis 2010;16(1):20–8.
113. McAllister BS. Stem cell-containing allograft matrix enhances periodontal regeneration: case presentations. Int J Periodontics Restorative Dent 2011;31(2): 149–55.
114. Koo S, Alshihri A, Karimbux NY, et al. Cellular allograft in the treatment of a severe periodontal intrabony defect: a case report. Clin Adv Periodontics 2012; 2(1):35–9.
115. Yamada Y, Nakamura S, Ito K, et al. Injectable bone tissue engineering using expanded mesenchymal stem cells. Stem Cells 2013;31(3):572–80.
116. Rosen PS. A case report on combination therapy using a composite allograft containing mesenchymal cells with an amnion-chorion barrier to treat a mandibular class III furcation. Clin Adv Periodontics 2013;3(2):64–9.
117. Aimetti M, Ferrarotti F, Cricenti L, et al. Autologous dental pulp stem cells in periodontal regeneration: a case report. Int J Periodontics Restorative Dent 2014; 34:S27–33.
118. Aimetti M, Ferrarotti F, Mariani GM, et al. Use of dental pulp stem cells/collagen sponge biocomplex in the treatment of non-contained intrabony defects: a case series. Clin Adv Periodontics 2015;5(2):104–9.
119. Baba S, Yamada Y, Komuro A, et al. Phase I/II trial of autologous bone marrow stem cell transplantation with a three-dimensional woven-fabric scaffold for periodontitis. Stem Cells Int 2016;2016:6205910.
120. Li Y, Zhao S, Nan X, et al. Repair of human periodontal bone defects by autologous grafting stem cells derived from inflammatory dental pulp tissues. Stem Cell Res Ther 2016;7:141.
121. Chen FM, Gao LN, Tian BM, et al. Treatment of periodontal intrabony defects using autologous periodontal ligament stem cells: a randomized clinical trial. Stem Cell Res Ther 2016;7:33.
122. KI V, Ryana H, Dalvi PJ. Autologous periodontal stem cell assistance in periodontal regeneration technique (SAI-PRT) in the treatment of periodontal intrabony defects: a case report with one-year follow-up. J Dent Res Dent Clin Dent Prospects 2017;11(2):123–6.
123. Aimetti M, Ferrarotti F, Gamba MN, et al. Regenerative treatment of periodontal intrabony defects using autologous dental pulp stem cells: a 1-year follow-up case series. Int J Periodontics Restorative Dent 2018;38(1):51–9.
124. Ferrarotti F, Romano F, Gamba MN, et al. Human intrabony defect regeneration with micrografts containing dental pulp stem cells: a randomized controlled clinical trial. J Clin Periodontol 2018;45(7):841–50.
125. Hernandez-Monjaraz B, Santiago-Osorio E, Ledesma-Martinez E, et al. Retrieval of a periodontally compromised tooth by allogeneic grafting of mesenchymal stem cells from dental pulp: a case report. J Int Med Res 2018;46(7):2983–93.
126. Shalini HS, Vandana KL. Direct application of autologous periodontal ligament stem cell niche in treatment of periodontal osseous defects: a randomized controlled trial. J Indian Soc Periodontol 2018;22(6):503–12.
127. Hernandez-Monjaraz B, Santiago-Osorio E, Ledesma-Martinez E, et al. Dental pulp mesenchymal stem cells as a treatment for periodontal disease in older adults. Stem Cells Int 2020;2020:8890873.

The Evolution of Surgical Techniques and Biomaterials for Periodontal Regeneration

Giorgio Pagni, DDS, MS[a], Lorenzo Tavelli, DDS, MS[b,c], Giulio Rasperini, DDS[a,*]

KEYWORDS

- Periodontal • Regeneration • Soft tissue grafting • Growth factor
- Gingival recession • Attachment loss

KEY POINTS

- Periodontal regenerative therapy has undergone several modifications over the year, including flap designs, barrier membranes, bone graft materials and biologic agents.
- Understanding the rationale for each surgical technique and biomaterial is crucial for planning the regenerative procedure.
- Minimally invasive flaps in combination with biologic agents can reduce the chance of papilla dehiscence/necrosis, post-operative morbidity and can enhance the regenerative outcomes.
- Recent techniques involve the regeneration of the intrabony defect together with the augmentation of the supracrestal soft tissue component.

INTRODUCTION

Just as osseointegration for endosseous dental implants, periodontal regeneration was a revolution for periodontal treatment. In an era in which bone resection was the only option to level unfavorable bone architecture for periodontal tissue maintenance, the possibility of leveling the defect by generating new attachments allowed for the proposal of several new techniques for maintaining the patients' natural dentition in health. Moreover, following Nyman and coworkers'[1] study on 1982 it was demonstrated that not only repair of the lost periodontal tissues was possible but also regeneration of

Conflict of interest and source of funding: The authors do not have any financial interests, either directly or indirectly, in the products or information enclosed in the article.
a Department of Biomedical, Surgical and Dental Sciences, University of Milan, Foundation IRCCS Ca' Granda Policlinic, Via della Commenda 12, Milan 20122, Italy; b Department of Periodontics, University of Michigan School of Dentistry, 1011 N University Avenue, Ann Arbor, MI 48109, USA; c Department of Oral Medicine, Infection, and Immunity, Division of Periodontology, Harvard School of Dental Medicine, 188 Longwood Avenue, Boston, MA 02115, USA
* Corresponding author. Via xx Settembre, 119 I-29100, Piacenza, Italy.
E-mail address: giulio.rasperini@unimi.it

the complete periodontal architecture with new bone, new cementum, and new connective tissue with perpendicularly oriented fibers was achievable.

The full potential of this at-the-time novel therapy is yet to be uncovered.

From flap design and suturing techniques to biomaterials for wound stabilization, from the concept of compartmentalization to that of blood clot stabilization, from scaffolding technologies to biological agents and growth factors to cell therapy our understanding of periodontal regeneration is constantly evolving.

THE EARLY STAGES

Nyman and coworkers'[1] report of periodontal tissue regeneration adopted an extended flap sutured over a millipore filter placed to act as a barrier membrane between the soft tissues and the root surface. The investigators applied the occlusive to prevent the migration of dentogingival epithelium and gingival connective tissue cells into the defect along the curetted root surface. Progenitor cells originating from the adjacent periodontal ligament (PDL) and alveolar bone were therefore enabled to colonize the blood clot and induce periodontal regeneration. After 3 months of healing histologic analysis revealed the formation of new attachment in coronal direction to a level 5 mm coronal to the alveolar bone crest. This article reported for the first time on a human histologic evidence of new bone and new cementum formation together with the regeneration of a periodontal ligament with perpendicularly oriented fibers.[1]

Earlier studies from Schallhorn and colleagues[2] adopted autogenous grafts for periodontal tissue regeneration, and other reports attempted to apically position the flaps to allow bone cells to populate the defect before epithelial cells could. Nevertheless, the radiographic filling of the intrabony defect due to the properties of the bone graft could not be considered an evidence of periodontal regeneration.[3] A preclinical study demonstrated that the healing of some procedures that were considered "regenerative" (including the modified Widman flap, with or without different bone grafts) occurred by repair, with the formation of long junctional epithelium.[4]

Later on, Melcher introduced the concept of compartmentalization, speculating that different cell populations "compete" to repopulate the periodontal defect. To obtain periodontal regeneration, cells migrating from the epithelium and connective tissue layers have to be excluded from the defect.[5] Based on this theory, it was demonstrated that barrier membranes can effectively favor the migration of cells from the periodontal ligament into the infrabony defect, resulting in a true regeneration of periodontal ligament, cementum, and alveolar bone.[1] Different barrier membranes were developed with the idea of allowing for new tissue formation inside the vertical periodontal defect. Expanded polytetrafluoroethylene (e-PTFE) membranes were porous nonresorbable membranes characterized by the presence of an open microstructured collar, designed to stop epithelial cell migration via contact inhibition, and a partially occlusive device developed to allow compartmentalization of the defect while allowing for nutrients to sustain the flap integrity. Five weeks after the surgery these membranes were removed. Absorbable membranes eliminated the need for this second intervention and proved their proficiency in several studies.

These approaches were called guided tissue regeneration where the word "guided" maintained that the barrier membrane had the ability to direct the regeneration of tissues.

Despite the encouraging results these approaches had several limitations.

Flap design was not optimized for regenerative approaches and the tendency was to use extended flaps thus decreasing the stability during wound healing. In the early stages of periodontal regeneration interdental tissues were often discarded, bone substitutes were used as scaffolds and membranes as barriers, but the ability to maintain primary wound closure required the release of the flap and was hindered by the lack of an adequate amount of soft tissue to cover the interproximal areas. Despite these limitations guided tissue regeneration (GTR) proved to be superior to open flap debridement in terms of clinical attachment level gain and probing depth reduction and superior to osseous resective surgery in terms of clinical attachment levels. These results were confirmed in the short term,[6–8] and long term-follow-up studies proved them to be stable even after 10 to 15 years.[9–12]

Compromised teeth that were once sacrificed to maintain a positive architecture could then be maintained, and clinical attachment could be gained to improve tooth prognosis.

Tissue engineering developed new materials to attempt to overcome some of the limitations of this approach to achieve more predictable results and faster and better tissue regeneration.

PAPILLA PRESERVATION FLAPS

The importance of defect isolation by occlusion membranes on tissue regeneration was questioned in several articles. In GTR, the formation of a long junctional epithelium as a consequence of periodontal repair as opposed to regeneration has been suggested to be more closely related to wound failure rather than to failure of defect isolation per se.[13,14] Several studies reported on the critical role of an uncomplicated adsorption, adhesion, and maturation of the fibrin clot at the tooth-mucogingival flap interface to achieve a new connective tissue attachment and to prevent the downgrowth of the junctional epithelium.[13–15]

In 1985, Takei and colleagues[16] suggested a new flap design called papilla preservation flap with the intent of preserving the interdental papilla via a buccal semilunar incision. The vertical defects were accessed elevating the flap, and the interdental tissues were preserved attached to the palatal flap. After debridment and bone grafting the flaps were sutured with external crossed mattress sutures. Despite the innovative approach described by this article this flap design was not adopted by many practitioners.[16]

Ten years later, in 1995, Cortellini and Tonetti[17] described the modified papilla preservation flap. In their approach the incision line was moved lingually and a double-layer internal mattress suture technique was described. The importance of maintaining flap stability started to become more preeminent, and an increased attention to the suturing technique was adopted.[17]

Soon after, in 1999, the simplified papilla preservation flap was described with the intent of allowing for interdental tissue maintenance even in areas with narrow interdental spaces (<2 mm).[18] The simplified papilla preservation flap was not as performing as the modified papilla preservation flap, although it could be used in more clinical scenarios and was simpler to perform, therefore it became more and more accepted in the periodontal community.

These flaps were described to be used in combination with xenogeneic bone substitutes and resorbable membranes, and the flaps had to be elevated to receive.

MINIMALLY INVASIVE FLAPS

In the same year the simplified papilla preservation flap was described Rasperini and coworkers[19] described the surgical technique for enamel matrix derivative (EMD). Three case reports documented flaps with reduced elevation adopted in combination with EMD alone in esthetic areas. A modified mattress suture was used. All cases showed complete radiographic bone fill and no gingival recession. Re-entry surgery demonstrated complete closure of the vertical defects.

For the first time it was demonstrated that the membrane could be avoided and more limited flap elevation could help wound healing in contained defects even in the absence of bone grafts.

This new understanding of wound healing biology switched the focus of the regenerative procedure from the compartmentalization concept proposed by Melcher and supported by Nyman and coworkers' case report to the blood clot stability concept.

In 2003, Wachtel and colleagues[20] reported on the use of minimally invasive flaps in combination with EMDs. Buccal and lingual sulcular incisions were performed with microsurgical blade, and the papilla above the periodontal defect was elevated using the modified papilla preservation technique.[20]

In 2007, Cortellini and Tonetti[21] proposed the minimally invasive surgical technique (MIST), a modification of the modifier papilla preservation flap designed to limit the mesiodistal flap extension and the coronoapical reflection to reduce the surgical trauma and increase flap stability and to be used in combination with the application of EMD in the treatment of isolated deep intrabony defects. The flap design was enhanced by the adoption of an operating microscope and microsurgical instruments. Thirteen cases were reported in this preliminary cohort study suggesting that excellent results could be achieved with low patient morbidity associated to the surgery.[21]

Another advancement in the surgical techniques was suggested by Trombelli and coworkers[22] with the single flap approach (SFA) first described in a case series report in an Italian paper and then in an international magazine the following year. Trombelli's intuition was that if the defect could be accessed and degranulated elevating just one flap either buccal or lingual to the incision line, the elevation of the other flap was unnecessary. By not elevating both flaps wound closure was easier and blood clot stability enhanced by the maintenance of transgingival fibers in the notelevated flap and by the improved anchorage of the elevated one to the former thanks to an accurate suturing technique. In the same journal Cortellini and Tonetti[23] further improved their MIST with the modified MIST, which again promoted the importance to elevate only the buccal flap while keeping the lingual one unelevated. In cases where the defect is not accessible from the buccal aspect, the investigators suggested not to use the modified version of the MIST.

These improved approaches to periodontal regeneration were diffused widely by many speakers in international meetings, although the technical difficulties and required attention to detail partially hindered their adoption by several periodontal schools that still preferred the guided tissue regeneration with extended flaps and membranes. Nevertheless, it should be noted that minimally invasive approaches cannot be adopted in all clinical scenarios.[24]

A specific clinical scenario that is at times encountered especially in the lower anterior mandible is represented by loss of attachment in teeth with particularly close root proximity. In such cases even an incision line as the simplified papilla preservation flap would cut through a very narrow papilla that would be difficult to suture and would anyway have a hard time maintaining its stability throughout the healing process. To reduce suffering of this fragile area the entire papilla preservation technique was developed.[25] This flap design makes use of a "J"-shaped vertical incision one tooth apart from the defect to be treated. The defect can be accessed avoiding cutting the papilla at all, and biological agents can be applied through this lateral access. Sutures are then only put on the vertical incision in an area that is well vascularized and has a tendency to heal with minimal complication thus maintaining excellent stability of the clot during wound healing.

By designing flaps specifically to boost the potential of periodontal regeneration new attachment was shown to be possibly formed even in severely compromised teeth with attachment loss to the apex, teeth considered hopeless just a few years before.[26] Despite being technique and operator sensitive and therefore not applicable in anybody's hands, the improvement in flap design had a tremendous impact on the possibility to preserve patients' natural dentition in health and function, which is eventually the primary goal of periodontal therapy.

COMBINED INTRABONY- AND SOFT TISSUE- REGENERATIVE APPROACHES

Some investigators suggested that periodontal regeneration could benefit from the use of flaps described for root coverage procedures.[27-29] Rasperini and colleagues[27] introduced the "soft tissue wall technique" for the regenerative treatment of noncontained intrabony defects. This technique involves a trapezoidal coronally advanced flap that is first stabilized with sling sutures and then with an internal mattress suture for achieving primary intention healing and closure of the papilla.[27]

Based on the claimed advantages of the tunnel technique for root coverage (high esthetic outcomes, blood supply, graft nutrition, and quick healing[30,31]), some techniques avoiding the incision of the papilla have been described.[25,32-34] In particular, Najafi and coworkers[34] suggested the use of modified vestibular incision subperiosteal tunnel access. On the other hand, Moreno Rodriguez and colleagues[32] claimed that a better access and clinical outcomes can be achieved if an apical horizontal incision is made in the buccal aspect of the alveolar mucosa (on cortical healthy bone) instead of at the interproximal area. The investigators showed that this nonincised papillae surgical approach was not only able to provide a significant improvement in clinical attachment level but also a significant recession reduction (0.25 ± 0.44 mm) and a coronal advancement of the tip of the papillae after 1 year (0.4 ± 0.5 mm).[33] This technique can also be combined with a connective tissue graft for the treatment of intrabony defects.[35]

Trombelli and colleagues[36] further demonstrated that adding a connective tissue graft can improve the outcomes of SFA, in terms of coronal position of the gingival margin and increase in soft tissue volume. Based on the connective tissue graft wall technique introduced for improving root coverage and clinical attachment level in RT3 gingival recessions,[37] Zucchelli and coworkers[38] proposed to use a connective tissue graft obtained from the de-epithelialization of a free gingival graft and stabilized on the buccal aspect of noncontained infrabony defects as a biological barrier for promoting, in combination with EMDs, periodontal regeneration.

BIOMATERIALS
Barrier Membranes

Periodontal regeneration started with the introduction of barrier membranes. Nonresorbable membranes include titanium foils and ePTFE with or without a titanium reinforcement. These membranes are able to maintain the space necessary for both periodontal and bone regeneration.[39] Nevertheless, the high incidence of membrane exposure and the necessity of an additional surgery for removing the membrane are the main drawback of these materials. These disadvantages led clinicians to explore the use of biodegradable membranes for periodontal regeneration. Resorbable membranes include polyesters (ie, polyglycolic acid, polylactic acid) and tissue-derived collagens.[40] Polymeric resorbable membranes maintain their maximum stability for about 14 days and then gradually lose their structural and mechanical properties within 1 month, but they have limited biocompatibility.[41,42] On the other hand, collagen membranes have a great biocompatibility and also poor mechanical properties.[40] Although some studies showed greater outcomes for nonresorbable membranes (when not exposed) compared with resorbable membranes,[43] only the latter are nowadays used for periodontal regeneration purposes. Indeed, the use of resorbable membranes is now supported by a larger evidence and increased experience levels.

Last, it has to be mentioned that e-PTFE membranes were replaced by high-density PTFE (d-PTFE) membranes, characterized by smaller pore size that may reduce the drawbacks of early membrane exposure. Nevertheless, d-PTFE membranes are mostly used in guided bone regeneration.[44]

Filling Materials

The rationale on the use of filling materials for periodontal regenerative procedures is mainly related to their scaffolding, space maintenance, and blood clot-stabilizing properties. Several filling materials have been used in periodontal regeneration, including autogenous bone grafts, xenografts, allografts, and synthetic bone grafts. Autogenous bone graft is the only bone filler that has osteogenic, osteoinductive, and osteoconductive properties at the same time.[44] Nevertheless, its harvesting often requires an additional surgical site with increased patient morbidity, and a significant remodeling has also been considered one of the main drawbacks of autogenous grafts.[44] On the other hand, the resorption rate of bone substitutes instead is quite slow.[45,46] In the regeneration of tooth-supporting structures, autologous grafts demonstrated high potential for periodontal growth,[47] but the current tendency of performing minimally invasive approaches limits the use of this scaffold material.

Nevertheless, according to a Bayesian network meta-analysis of Tu and coworkers,[48] combination therapies performed better than single therapies, with GTR and bone grafts showing the greatest defect fill. However, it has to be mentioned that the additional benefits of combination therapies were considered small.[48]

Last, scaffold technology has rapidly evolved in the last years. Creating personalized three-dimensional printed polymeric scaffolds may represent the future direction of periodontal regeneration.[49] Our group described the first-in-human application use of a three-dimensional bioprinted scaffolding matrix to treat a periodontal defect.[50] The scaffold was made of polycaprolactone biomaterial to custom fit the osseous architecture of a patient presenting with a large, localized periodontal osseous defect of critical size. This defect could not have been treated with traditional scaffolding approaches. The treated area remained covered and showed evidence of early clinical reattachment.[50]

Biological Agents

Enamel matrix proteins are deposited on the developing tooth roots before the formation of the cementum.[51,52] It has been shown that EMDs obtained from porcine fetal tooth biomimetically stimulate cementogenesis by enhancing proliferation and migration of periodontal ligament cells and osteoblasts, mimicking the natural process of tooth development.[53–55] A recent review summarizing the properties and outcomes of EMDs highlighted the large evidence supporting its efficacy in periodontal regeneration. Nevertheless, it is still unclear whether this biological agent would benefit from the utilization of carrier systems.[54]

Platelet-derived growth factor-BB (PDGF-BB) is one of most investigated growth factors in periodontal tissue engineering; its properties of promoting bone, cementum, and PDL regeneration have been confirmed in animal and clinical studies.[56–59] This growth factor is able to enhance the proliferation and chemotaxis of cells from the periodontal ligament and alveolar bone cells.[57,60–62] A large multicenter randomized controlled trial demonstrated the safety and efficacy of PDGF-BB in periodontal regeneration, with significantly higher clinical attachment gain and bone fill compared with the carrier alone.[59] Interestingly, no barrier membranes were used in combination with PDGF-BB.[59]

Other biological agents include platelet concentrates and fibroblast growth factor.[63] There is limited (and controversial) evidence regarding the role of platelet concentrates for periodontal regeneration.[64,65] Although some initial promising results have been reported for the fibroblast growth factor,[5,66] more studies are necessary to evaluate the regenerative properties of this biological agent.

CONCLUDING REMARKS

We reviewed here the evolution of periodontal regenerative approaches over a period of almost 40 years. This article highlights the revolution that periodontal regeneration allowed in periodontal therapy.

Periodontal regeneration allows for maintenance of teeth that could not be preserved when open flaps and osseous resective surgery were the only options to re-create a positive architecture that is easy to clean. This is clearly a revolution not only because of the many teeth we can now maintain but also because it determines a switch in an important paradigm of periodontal therapy. The definition of periodontal disease was once that of gingival inflammation causing an irreversible loss of clinical attachment level. The classification of periodontal disease itself differentiates the stage of the disease according to loss of interproximal attachment. We recently published an article highlighting how by regenerating interproximal attachment we can now reverse the periodontal condition of our patients and bring them back to a less-severe stage of periodontal disease.[28]

Several advanced tissue engineering approaches are being studied, which may keep evolving our understanding and ability to regenerate lost tissues.

Unfortunately, the evolution of periodontal regeneration led to enhanced difficulty of some of the proposed techniques requiring not only a basic periodontal setting but also the availability of operating microscopes, scaffolding biomaterials, and biological agents increasing the overhead and making the logistic of these treatments more complicated. These drawbacks are reducing the diffusion of such techniques making them accessible just to a limited patient population while many practitioners choose to rely on the least technique-sensitive and more predictable traditional approach. It is imperative that the periodontal community sticks together and actively puts its maximum effort toward increasing the awareness on the potential of periodontal regeneration in the maintenance of natural dentition, especially in the education of younger generations of periodontal specialists. New advancements are continuously evolving our knowledge of the biological mechanisms lying behind the regeneration of a complex structure such as the periodontal ligament and related tissues. By improving our knowledge, we are able to provide enhanced possibilities for the treatment of periodontal patients. We cannot walk back to earlier stages. We must only look forward.

CLINICS CARE POINTS

- Several techniques have been progressively introduced for periodontal regeneration.
- While at the beginning the surgical techniques for periodontal regeneration were aimed at preserving the integrity of the papilla and providing good visibility and access for utilizing barrier membranes, the introduction of biologic agents has allowed for minimally invasive surgical approaches.

- Nowadays, a large variety of bone graft materials, collagen membrane and biologic agents is available on the market and clinicians should choose the most appropriate biomaterial(s) based on the characteristics of the defect.
- Utilizing soft tissue grafts at the same time of the periodontal regenerative therapy can further enhance the interproximal attachment gain and esthetic outcomes, which is particularly crucial for infrabony defects in the esthetic area.

REFERENCES

1. Nyman S, Lindhe J, Karring T, et al. New attachment following surgical treatment of human periodontal disease. J Clin Periodontol 1982;9:290–6.
2. Schallhorn RG, Hiatt WH, Boyce W. Iliac transplants in periodontal therapy. J Periodontol 1970;41:566–80.
3. Rosen PS, Reynolds MA, Bowers GM. The treatment of intrabony defects with bone grafts. Periodontol 2000 2000;22:88–103.
4. Caton J, Nyman S, Zander H. Histometric evaluation of periodontal surgery. II. Connective tissue attachment levels after four regenerative procedures. J Clin Periodontol 1980;7:224–31.
5. Cochran DL, Oh TJ, Mills MP, et al. A Randomized Clinical Trial Evaluating rh-FGF-2/beta-TCP in Periodontal Defects. J Dent Res 2016;95:523–30.
6. Esposito M, Grusovin MG, Papanikolaou N, et al. Enamel matrix derivative (Emdogain) for periodontal tissue regeneration in intrabony defects. A Cochrane systematic review. Eur J Oral Implantol 2009;2:247–66.
7. Needleman I, Tucker R, Giedrys-Leeper E, et al. Guided tissue regeneration for periodontal intrabony defects–a Cochrane Systematic Review. Periodontol 2000 2005;37:106–23.
8. Trombelli L, Heitz-Mayfield LJ, Needleman I, et al. A systematic review of graft materials and biological agents for periodontal intraosseous defects. J Clin Periodontol 2002;29(Suppl 3):117–35 [discussion: 160–2].
9. Nickles K, Ratka-Kruger P, Neukranz E, et al. Open flap debridement and guided tissue regeneration after 10 years in infrabony defects. J Clin Periodontol 2009; 36:976–83.
10. Pretzl B, Kim TS, Steinbrenner H, et al. Guided tissue regeneration with bioabsorbable barriers III 10-year results in infrabony defects. J Clin Periodontol 2009;36:349–56.
11. Sculean A, Kiss A, Miliauskaite A, et al. Ten-year results following treatment of intra-bony defects with enamel matrix proteins and guided tissue regeneration. J Clin Periodontol 2008;35:817–24.
12. Silvestri M, Rasperini G, Milani S. 120 infrabony defects treated with regenerative therapy: long-term results. J Periodontol 2011;82:668–75.
13. Wikesjo UM, Nilveus RE, Selvig KA. Significance of early healing events on periodontal repair: a review. J Periodontol 1992;63:158–65.
14. Wikesjo UM, Selvig KA. Periodontal wound healing and regeneration. Periodontol 2000 1999;19:21–39.
15. Hiatt WH, Stallard RE, Butler ED, et al. Repair following mucoperiosteal flap surgery with full gingival retention. J Periodontol 1968;39:11–6.
16. Takei HH, Han TJ, Carranza FA Jr, et al. Flap technique for periodontal bone implants. Papilla preservation technique. J Periodontol 1985;56:204–10.

17. Cortellini P, Prato GP, Tonetti MS. The modified papilla preservation technique. A new surgical approach for interproximal regenerative procedures. J Periodontol 1995;66:261–6.
18. Cortellini P, Prato GP, Tonetti MS. The simplified papilla preservation flap. A novel surgical approach for the management of soft tissues in regenerative procedures. Int J Periodontics Restorative Dent 1999;19:589–99.
19. Rasperini G, Ricci G, Silvestri M. Surgical technique for treatment of infrabony defects with enamel matrix derivative (Emdogain): 3 case reports. Int J Periodontics Restorative Dent 1999;19:578–87.
20. Wachtel H, Schenk G, Bohm S, et al. Microsurgical access flap and enamel matrix derivative for the treatment of periodontal intrabony defects: a controlled clinical study. J Clin Periodontol 2003;30:496–504.
21. Cortellini P, Tonetti MS. A minimally invasive surgical technique with an enamel matrix derivative in the regenerative treatment of intra-bony defects: a novel approach to limit morbidity. J Clin Periodontol 2007;34:87–93.
22. Trombelli L, Farina R, Franceschetti G, et al. Single-flap approach with buccal access in periodontal reconstructive procedures. J Periodontol 2009;80:353–60.
23. Cortellini P, Tonetti MS. Improved wound stability with a modified minimally invasive surgical technique in the regenerative treatment of isolated interdental intrabony defects. J Clin Periodontol 2009;36:157–63.
24. Cortellini P, Tonetti MS. Clinical concepts for regenerative therapy in intrabony defects. Periodontol 2000 2015;68:282–307.
25. Aslan S, Buduneli N, Cortellini P. Entire Papilla Preservation Technique: A Novel Surgical Approach for Regenerative Treatment of Deep and Wide Intrabony Defects. Int J Periodontics Restorative Dent 2017;37:227–33.
26. Cortellini P, Stalpers G, Mollo A, et al. Periodontal regeneration versus extraction and prosthetic replacement of teeth severely compromised by attachment loss to the apex: 5-year results of an ongoing randomized clinical trial. J Clin Periodontol 2011;38:915–24.
27. Rasperini G, Acunzo R, Barnett A, et al. The soft tissue wall technique for the regenerative treatment of non-contained infrabony defects: a case series. Int J Periodontics Restorative Dent 2013;33:e79–87.
28. Rasperini G, Tavelli L, Barootchi S, et al. Interproximal attachment gain: The challenge of periodontal regeneration. J Periodontol 2020. https://doi.org/10.1002/JPER.20-0587.
29. Zucchelli G, De Sanctis M. A novel approach to minimizing gingival recession in the treatment of vertical bony defects. J Periodontol 2008;79:567–74.
30. Tavelli L, Barootchi S, Nguyen TVN, et al. Efficacy of tunnel technique in the treatment of localized and multiple gingival recessions: A systematic review and meta-analysis. J Periodontol 2018;89:1075–90.
31. Zuhr O, Rebele SF, Schneider D, et al. Tunnel technique with connective tissue graft versus coronally advanced flap with enamel matrix derivative for root coverage: a RCT using 3D digital measuring methods. Part I. Clinical and patient-centred outcomes. J Clin Periodontol 2014;41:582–92.
32. Moreno Rodriguez JA, Ortiz Ruiz AJ, Caffesse RG. Periodontal reconstructive surgery of deep intraosseous defects using an apical approach. Non-incised papillae surgical approach (NIPSA): A retrospective cohort study. J Periodontol 2019a;90:454–64.
33. Moreno Rodriguez JA, Ortiz Ruiz AJ, Caffesse RG. Supra-alveolar attachment gain in the treatment of combined intra-suprabony periodontal defects by non-incised papillae surgical approach. J Clin Periodontol 2019b;46:927–36.

34. Najafi B, Kheirieh P, Torabi A, et al. Periodontal Regenerative Treatment of Intrab-ony Defects in the Esthetic Zone Using Modified Vestibular Incision Subperiosteal Tunnel Access (M-VISTA). Int J Periodontics Restorative Dent 2018;38:e9–16.
35. Moreno Rodriguez JA, Ortiz Ruiz AJ, Zamora GP, et al. Connective Tissue Grafts with Nonincised Papillae Surgical Approach for Periodontal Reconstruction in Noncontained Defects. Int J Periodontics Restorative Dent 2019c;39:781–7.
36. Trombelli L, Simonelli A, Minenna L, et al. Effect of a Connective Tissue Graft in Combination With a Single Flap Approach in the Regenerative Treatment of Intra-osseous Defects. J Periodontol 2017;88:348–56.
37. Zucchelli G, Mazzotti C, Tirone F, et al. The connective tissue graft wall technique and enamel matrix derivative to improve root coverage and clinical attachment levels in Miller Class IV gingival recession. Int J Periodontics Restorative Dent 2014;34:601–9.
38. Zucchelli G, Mounssif I, Marzadori M, et al. Connective Tissue Graft Wall Tech-nique and Enamel Matrix Derivative for the Treatment of Infrabony Defects: Case Reports. Int J Periodontics Restorative Dent 2017;37:673–81.
39. Polimeni G, Koo KT, Qahash M, et al. Prognostic factors for alveolar regeneration: effect of a space-providing biomaterial on guided tissue regeneration. J Clin Pe-riodontol 2004;31:725–9.
40. Bottino MC, Thomas V, Schmidt G, et al. Recent advances in the development of GTR/GBR membranes for periodontal regeneration–a materials perspective. Dent Mater 2012;28:703–21.
41. Gentile P, Chiono V, Tonda-Turo C, et al. Polymeric membranes for guided bone regeneration. Biotechnol J 2011;6:1187–97.
42. Milella E, Ramires PA, Brescia E, et al. Physicochemical, mechanical, and biolog-ical properties of commercial membranes for GTR. J Biomed Mater Res 2001;58: 427–35.
43. Tal H, Kozlovsky A, Artzi Z, et al. Cross-linked and non-cross-linked collagen bar-rier membranes disintegrate following surgical exposure to the oral environment: a histological study in the cat. Clin Oral Implants Res 2008;19:760–6.
44. Ausenda F, Rasperini G, Acunzo R, et al. New Perspectives in the Use of Bioma-terials for Periodontal Regeneration. Materials (Basel) 2019;12. https://doi.org/10. 3390/ma12132197.
45. Amerio P, Vianale G, Reale M, et al. The effect of deproteinized bovine bone on osteoblast growth factors and proinflammatory cytokine production. Clin Oral Im-plants Res 2010;21:650–5.
46. Rasperini G, Canullo L, Dellavia C, et al. Socket grafting in the posterior maxilla reduces the need for sinus augmentation. Int J Periodontics Restorative Dent 2010;30:265–73.
47. Verdugo F, D'Addona A. Long-term stable periodontal regeneration by means of autologous bone grafting in patients with severe periodontitis. Int J Periodontics Restorative Dent 2012;32:157–64.
48. Tu YK, Needleman I, Chambrone L, et al. A Bayesian network meta-analysis on comparisons of enamel matrix derivatives, guided tissue regeneration and their combination therapies. J Clin Periodontol 2012;39:303–14.
49. Rios HF, Lin Z, Oh B, et al. Cell- and gene-based therapeutic strategies for peri-odontal regenerative medicine. J Periodontol 2011;82:1223–37.
50. Rasperini G, Pilipchuk SP, Flanagan CL, et al. 3D-printed Bioresorbable Scaffold for Periodontal Repair. J Dent Res 2015;94:153S–7S.

51. Lindskog S, Hammarstrom L. Formation of intermediate cementum. III: 3H-tryptophan and 3H-proline uptake into the epithelial root sheath of Hertwig in vitro. J Craniofac Genet Dev Biol 1982;2:171–7.
52. Slavkin HC, Bessem C, Fincham AG, et al. Human and mouse cementum proteins immunologically related to enamel proteins. Biochim Biophys Acta 1989; 991:12–8.
53. Hoang AM, Oates TW, Cochran DL. In vitro wound healing responses to enamel matrix derivative. J Periodontol 2000;71:1270–7.
54. Miron RJ, Sculean A, Cochran DL, et al. Twenty years of enamel matrix derivative: the past, the present and the future. J Clin Periodontol 2016;43:668–83.
55. Yoneda S, Itoh D, Kuroda S, et al. The effects of enamel matrix derivative (EMD) on osteoblastic cells in culture and bone regeneration in a rat skull defect. J Periodontal Res 2003;38:333–42.
56. Camelo M, Nevins ML, Schenk RK, et al. Periodontal regeneration in human Class II furcations using purified recombinant human platelet-derived growth factor-BB (rhPDGF-BB) with bone allograft. Int J Periodontics Restorative Dent 2003;23: 213–25.
57. Cho MI, Lin WL, Genco RJ. Platelet-derived growth factor-modulated guided tissue regenerative therapy. J Periodontol 1995;66:522–30.
58. Lynch SE, Williams RC, Polson AM, et al. A combination of platelet-derived and insulin-like growth factors enhances periodontal regeneration. J Clin Periodontol 1989;16:545–8.
59. Nevins M, Giannobile WV, McGuire MK, et al. Platelet-derived growth factor stimulates bone fill and rate of attachment level gain: results of a large multicenter randomized controlled trial. J Periodontol 2005;76:2205–15.
60. Dennison DK, Vallone DR, Pinero GJ, et al. Differential effect of TGF-beta 1 and PDGF on proliferation of periodontal ligament cells and gingival fibroblasts. J Periodontol 1994;65:641–8.
61. Matsuda N, Lin WL, Kumar NM, et al. Mitogenic, chemotactic, and synthetic responses of rat periodontal ligament fibroblastic cells to polypeptide growth factors in vitro. J Periodontol 1992;63:515–25.
62. Park JB, Matsuura M, Han KY, et al. Periodontal regeneration in class III furcation defects of beagle dogs using guided tissue regenerative therapy with platelet-derived growth factor. J Periodontol 1995;66:462–77.
63. Tavelli L, McGuire MK, Zucchelli G, et al. Biologics-based regenerative technologies for periodontal soft tissue engineering. J Periodontol 2020;91:147–54.
64. Castro AB, Meschi N, Temmerman A, et al. Regenerative potential of leucocyte- and platelet-rich fibrin. Part A: intra-bony defects, furcation defects and periodontal plastic surgery. A systematic review and meta-analysis. J Clin Periodontol 2017;44:67–82.
65. Miron RJ, Zucchelli G, Pikos MA, et al. Use of platelet-rich fibrin in regenerative dentistry: a systematic review. Clin Oral Investig 2017;21:1913–27.
66. Saito A, Bizenjima T, Takeuchi T, et al. Treatment of intrabony periodontal defects using rhFGF-2 in combination with deproteinized bovine bone mineral or rhFGF-2 alone: A 6-month randomized controlled trial. J Clin Periodontol 2019;46:332–41.

Soft Tissue Regeneration at Natural Teeth

Raluca Cosgarea, PhD, DDS, PD[a,b,c], Alpdogan Kantarci, DDS, PhD[d],
Andreas Stavropoulos, DDS, PhD, Dr. Odont.[e], Nicole Arweiler, DDS, PhD[b],
Anton Sculean, DMD, MS, PhD[f,*]

KEYWORDS

- Gingival recessions • Teeth • Recession coverage • Coronally advanced flap
- Modified coronally advanced tunnel

KEY POINTS

- The coronally advanced flap and tunnel are the most predictable techniques for the treatment of single and multiple gingival recessions.
- So far, long-term results for the coronally advanced flap with or without a connective tissue graft provide evidence for long-term stability with minor relapses.
- Biooogics and soft tissue replacement materials may additionally improve the clinical outcomes or may be used as an alternative to autogenous grafts.

INTRODUCTION

Gingival recession (GR) is a frequent clinical feature affecting most of the adult population[1–3] with an incidence of about 54% in young adults (26–35 years) and about 100% in middle-elderly adults (36–45 years).[4] GR is defined as the apical displacement of the gingival margin while exposing a portion of the root surface.[5] Various predisposing and/or causative factors may induce the appearance of GR, such as traumatic tooth brushing, plaque-induced inflammation, periodontitis[6,7] or viruses,[8] inadequate dental procedures invading the biologic width,[9] inadequate tooth alignment or other anatomic or periodontal features,[10] presence of muscle insertions close to the gingival margin,[11] lack of an adequate band of keratinized/attached gingiva,[12] reduced buccal-lingual thickness of the alveolar bone plate,[13] orthodontic tooth movement, or oral jewelry.[5,14] The presence of GR is regularly linked to aesthetic

[a] Department of Periodontology, Operative and Preventive Dentistry, University of Welschnonnenstr. 17, 53125 Bonn, Bonn, Germany; [b] Department of Periodontology and Peri-Implant Diseases, Philipps University of Marburg, Georg-Voigt. Str. 3, Marburg 35039, Germany; [c] Department of Prosthetic Dentistry, University Iuliu Hatieganu Cluj-Napoca, Str. Clinicilor nr 32, Cluj-Napoca 400056, Romania; [d] Forsyth Institute, 245 First Street, Cambridge, MA 02142, USA; [e] Department of Periodontology, University of Malmö, Carl Gustafs väg 34, 214 21 Malmö, Sweden; [f] Department of Periodontology, University of Bern, Freiburgstrasse, 7, Bern CH-3010, Switzerland
* Corresponding address.
E-mail address: anton.sculean@zmk.unibe.ch

Dent Clin N Am 66 (2022) 87–101
https://doi.org/10.1016/j.cden.2021.09.001
0011-8532/22/© 2021 Elsevier Inc. All rights reserved.

impairment, tooth hypersensitivity, and root caries, and may hinder an optimal self-performed oral hygiene leading to plaque accumulation and further tissue loss.[12,15–17]

Successful treatment of GR aims at restoring the lost periodontal tissues by achieving complete root coverage with optimal tissue integration, scar-free tissue blending, and physiologic clinical probing pocket depths. Thus, periodontal plastic surgical procedures with clinically predictable results for root coverage are indicated. At the beginning of the twentieth century, the use of pedicle gingival grafts or free gingival grafts (FGG) were first described by Younger (1902), Harlan (1906), and Rosenthal (1981)[18] for the surgical treatment of GR. Later, further surgical approaches, such as coronally advanced flaps (CAFs), coronally advanced tunnel flaps, laterally repositioned flaps alone or combined with FGG, or subepithelial connective tissue grafts (CTG) were presented as successful surgical techniques to improve recession depth, clinical attachment level, and width of keratinized tissue.[19–27]

Although the choice for the optimal surgical technique is still debatable, it is unequivocal that the additional use of a CTG represents the gold standard by providing the highest probability for complete root coverage with the greatest aesthetic results.[28–30] The combination with other biomaterials of various origins, such as acellular dermal matrix (ADM), xenogenic collagen matrices (XCM), enamel matrix derivatives (EMD), hyaluronic acid (HA), or platelet-rich fibrin (PRF), has also been investigated in this context.[31–40]

This narrative review provides an overview on the clinical outcomes and stability in time of the best-documented surgical techniques and biomaterials used for coverage of single and multiple GRs.

BIOLOGIC BACKGROUND

The healing process after soft tissue grafting has been extensively described in various animal and human histologic studies.[41–47] The healing and revascularization of an FGG was described in a histologic study in monkeys.[46] Three healing phases were recognized. First, an initial phase (0–3 days), where the graft was separated by the periosteum by a thin fibrin layer, accompanied by degeneration of the epithelium and desquamation of the outer layers. The following 4 to 11 days a revascularization phase was observed, characterized by minimal resorption of the alveolar bone, fibroblast proliferation in the graft-periosteum region, vascularization and capillary ingrowth at the base of the graft, and formation of an epithelial layer from the adjacent tissues over the graft. Thereafter, in the third phase, the maturation phase (11–42 days), the epithelium layer thickens and by the 28th day is keratinized. Meanwhile, the connective tissue increases in its density and gets poorer in vascular vessels. Similar histologic descriptions were reported by other authors,[41,42,48] emphasizing additionally that grafts placed onto the periosteum seem to have a better initial adaptation and graft nourishment as opposed to those placed directly onto the bone. Additionally, the latter ones seem to be characterized by wider degenerative changes and delayed epithelialization. Nonetheless, by the 28th healing day, in both situations (graft placed directly onto the bone, or onto the periosteum) the tissue seems to be keratinized.[41,42,48]

Soft tissue maturation after grafting, irrespective of the graft type (CTG or FGG) is accompanied by a significant tissue shrinkage, between 25% and 45%.[43–45,47,49] It was also described that thicker grafts provide less shrinkage but a more delayed revascularization.[43,45,49]

In a series of histologic animal studies, it was determined that the specificity of the epithelium (clinical and structural features) is genetically determined rather than the result of functional adaptation.[50] Additionally, it has been shown that even after complete excision of the keratinized tissue at teeth, a new band of attached gingiva will be formed.[51-53] Further histologic evidence exists related to the key role of the gingival connective tissue in genetically determining the specificity of the epithelia.[54] It has been additionally shown in animal and human studies, that the granulation tissue that proliferates from the periodontal ligament and the supra-alveolar connective tissue leads to formation of a keratinized tissue, whereas that originating from the alveolar mucosa leads to a nonkeratinized mucosa.[55,56]

Another biologically and clinically relevant aspect when using CTGs for keratinization purposes, is the depth of the donor tissue layer: possible differences between superficial and deep connective tissue layers seem to exist. Evaluations using histology, immunofluorescence, and gel electrophoresis provided evidence that CTGs from deep layers lead to a tissue containing keratinized and nonkeratinized characteristics. However, grafts originating from superficial layers (epithelial CTGs) always provide histologic and biochemical features of a keratinized mucosa.[57] Based on these findings and further human evidence,[58-60] the authors concluded that deep palatal CTGs may have a poorer potential to induce keratinization as opposed to connective tissues situated in immediate epithelial vicinity.

Taken together, the results of the previously mentioned studies indicate that keratinization is induced from granulation tissue originating from periodontal ligament or from connective tissue initially covered by keratinized epithelium; consequently, this indicates for the use of a palatal CTG in clinical situations with GR and/or with lack of keratinized tissue.

SURGICAL THERAPY FOR SINGLE RECESSIONS

The ultimate goal of surgical root coverage procedures is the complete root coverage with optimal color and texture blending of the covering tissue.[61,62] Numerous root coverage procedures including pedicle flaps, FGGs, laterally positioned flaps, double pedicle flaps, and various forms of CAFs or tunnels have been described.[63,64]

One of the most reliable and best investigated surgical approaches for single recessions is the CAF.[61,65-68] With CAF, the soft tissue apical to the recession is coronally advanced to accomplish root coverage, as follows.[69] Mesially and distally to the recession, two beveled horizontal incisions (about 3 mm) are made; these are located at a distance from the tip of the anatomic papillae that equals the recession depth plus 1 mm. From the horizontal incisions, two beveled vertical incisions are performed into the alveolar mucosa resulting in a trapezoidal flap with two surgical papillae. This is elevated as a split flap in the papilla region, followed by a full-thickness elevation of the tissue apical to the recession until the mucogingival junction and 3 mm of the apical bone is exposed; thereafter, a second split-flap is raised apically until tension-free, passive coronal flap advancement so that it is possible to completely cover the recession coronally to the cementoenamel junction (CEJ). For this, all muscle insertions attached to the flap are cut. Next, the vestibular sites of the anatomic papillae are de-epithelialized coronally to the initial horizontal incisions to obtain a connective tissue bed where the surgical papillae will be sutured. Finally, the flap is sutured with single interrupted sutures, oriented from the flap to the adjacent soft tissue in apicocoronal direction. At the apical end of the vertical incisions, the flap is fixed with two periosteal sutures, so as to minimize any coronal flap movements. The surgical papillae are adapted to the anatomic papillae by means of sling sutures allowing a tight and precise flap adaptation to the crown of the tooth.[69]

In CAF and most of the previously mentioned surgical procedures, a split flap approach is adopted, which sometimes, specifically in clinical situations with a thin gingiva, may be difficult to perform risking flap perforation and possible graft necrosis. To minimize these risks, the modified coronally advanced tunnel (MCAT),[70] a modification of the tunnel procedure, and the laterally closed tunnel (LCT)[71] with either CTG with or without biologics, such as EMD or HA, or soft tissue replacement materials have been described.[32,33,38–40,71,72]

In MCAT, a mucoperiosteal flap is prepared by means of tunneling instruments while maintaining the interdental papillae intact.[72] The mucoperiosteal tunnel is then extended apically and laterally into a partial thickness flap while all attaching muscles and inserting collagen fibers are sectioned and released from the inner aspect of the tunnel flap. The interdental papillae are gently undermined with specially designed tunneling knives paying special attention not to rupture or perforate the flap and/or the papillae. Subsequently, the prepared tunnel flap is passively advanced coronally. In cases with thin phenotype a CTG is indicated. The CTG is harvested from the palate and then pulled in the tunnel using single or mattress sutures. The graft is fixed at the inner aspect of the tunnel flap mesially and distally, and tightly adapted at the CEJ by a sling suture. Finally, the tunnel flap is moved coronally using sling sutures to completely cover the graft and the recession, thus creating an excellent environment for wound healing.[72]

In cases with deep isolated anterior mandibular GRs LCT may be indicated.[71] Similar to MCAT, in LCT, a mucoperiosteal pouch is prepared using tunneling instruments and mobilized extensively mesially, distally, and apically beyond the mucogingival junction to attain passive lateral displacement of the pouch margins and cover completely/the greatest part of the exposed root. To achieve tension-free mobilization, all muscle insertions and fibers must be released from the inner aspect of the pouch. Interdental papillae are carefully undermined with tunneling knives and microsurgical blades taking special care not to disrupt them (**Fig. 1**A–D). Thereafter, a CTG harvested from the palate is pulled and fixed at the inner aspect of the pouch using single or mattress sutures. Subsequently, the CTG is tightly adapted at the CEJ level by means of a sling suture (**Fig. 1**E, F). Then the pouch margins are carefully pulled

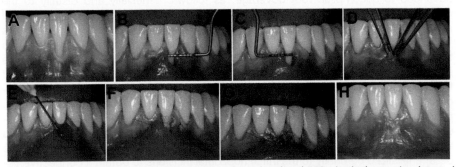

Fig. 1. (A) Preoperative situation depicting a deep, localized RT2 gingival recession located labially at tooth 31 (Case Anton Sculean). (B) Prepared mesial tunnel. (C) Prepared distal tunnel. (D) Tension-free mobilization of the tunnel allowing complete coverage of the exposed root surface. (E) Application of hyaluronic acid to enhance periodontal and soft tissue healing. (F) Subepithelial CTG fixed at the CEJ. (G) Lateral closure of the tunnel enabling a tension-free postoperative situation. An almost complete coverage of the CTG is visible. (H) Clinical outcome indicates an excellent recession coverage and substantial gain of attached, keratinized soft tissue. Please note the absence of scar tissue and the natural tissue blending.

together over the graft and sutured with single interrupted sutures allowing a tension-free coverage and enabling an excellent healing (**Fig. 1**G, H).

SURGICAL THERAPY FOR MULTIPLE ADJACENT GINGIVAL RECESSIONS

Surgical treatment of multiple adjacent gingival recessions (MAGR) represents a challenging clinical situation. Treatment of MAGR supposes the coverage of multiple adjacent recessions of various depths and widths, with frequently different tooth positions, shallow vestibulum, and large avascular surfaces to be covered.

Three major surgical techniques have been shown to be successful for treating MAGR[73]: (1) CAF with two vertical incisions mesially and distally, (2) the modified version of CAF without releasing incisions,[74] and (3) the MCAT. Irrespective of the used technique, it seems that for all types of recessions (Miller I-IV, respectively, RT1, 2, 3) the addition of a CTG provides the best aesthetic results and is the most predictable method for achieving complete root coverage.[28–30,75–77]

Similarly as in CAF for single GRs, CAF applied in MAGR defects starts with a horizontal incision in the papilla area continuous with intrasulcular incisions that extend to one tooth more mesially and distally from the recessions creating several surgical papillae.[74] Thereafter, a split-full-split thickness envelope flap is prepared in the entire recession area and all inserting muscle fibers are released to achieve passive mobilization over the exposed root surfaces. Additionally, a CTG may be sutured with resorbable sutures to the papillae and periosteum over the exposed root surfaces and at the level of the CEJ. Finally, the flap is tightly adapted over the CTG and the exposed root surfaces with sling sutures. After previous de-epithelization of the anatomic papillae, the newly formed surgical papillae are sutured at the tip of the anatomic papillae.[74]

Another technique with promising results that has been intensively tested in the last decade is MCAT.[72,78] After intrasulcular incisions, a mucoperiosteal flap is raised using tunneling knives beyond the mucogingival junction and further extended as split flap apically and laterally. All inserting muscle and collagen fibers are released from the inner aspect of the tunnel flap to achieve passive (tension-free) complete coronal displacement over the exposed root surfaces. The interdental papillae are also carefully undermined to allow a CTG or a soft tissue replacement material to be pulled in the tunnel and fixed with mattress and sling sutures at the inner aspect of the tunnel and at the CEJ. Finally, the tunnel is coronally advanced to completely cover the graft/membrane and fixed with sling sutures to the teeth (**Figs. 2** and **3**).

Several short- and long-term studies pointed out that the additional use of a CTG to CAF is more effective and predictable in achieving complete root coverage compared with CAF alone in single and multiple recessions.[14,29,61,79–81] Moreover, it seems that the addition of CTG provided not only long-term stability but also greater increase in keratinized tissue.[82–84]

SOFT TISSUE BIOMATERIALS AND SUBSTITUTES

The adjunctive use of a CTG in surgical GR coverage has been repeatedly proven to show the best results in terms of complete root coverage, recession reduction, and increase in tissue thickness and attached/keratinized gingiva.[28–30,75–77] Nonetheless, in cases where a longer CTG is needed, graft prelevation becomes sometimes difficult, especially in cases with a thin palatal tissue, which in turn may increase patient morbidity and the risk for postsurgical complications. Most of the complications associated with soft tissue grafting are related to the donor site.[85–87] Harvesting of a free epithelial CTG may result in more severe complications, such as excessive

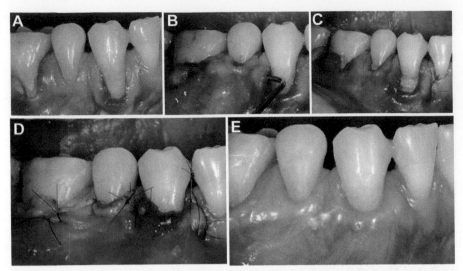

Fig. 2. (*A*) Preoperative view depicting the presence of multiple, adjacent gingival recessions located in the lower right quadrant. An inflamed gingiva is clearly visible because of difficulties in performing adequate oral hygiene measures (Case Anton Sculean). (*B*) Prepared tunnel. (*C*) Fixed CTG. (*D*) Coronally advanced and sutured tunnel to cover the recessions and the CTG. (*E*) The clinical outcome demonstrates complete root coverage and an increase in soft tissue thickness without tissue formation facilitating proper plaque control.

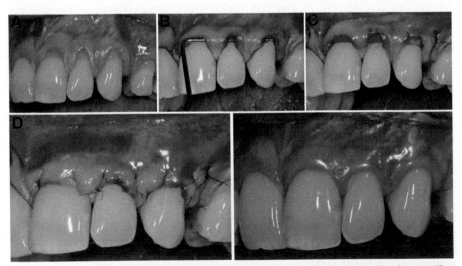

Fig. 3. (*A*) Preoperative view illustrating the presence of RT1 MAGR located in the maxillary anterior area. (*B*) Prepared tunnel. (*C*) A porcine ADM was pulled in the tunnel and fixed to the CEJ with sling sutures. (*D*) The tunnel was advanced coronally and sutured to completely cover the recessions and the ADM. (*E*) At 2 years postoperatively, the clinical outcome indicates complete coverage of all treated recessions.

hemorrhage, postoperative bone exposure, painful open palatal wound, and chewing discomfort compared with harvesting of a subepithelial CTG. It has been reported that mucogingival surgery including harvesting of epithelial CTGs was associated with 3.5 times more pain compared with osseous surgery and six times more pain compared with recession coverage.[85]

Because the infection rate following soft tissue grafting is low, the routine administration of systemic antibiotics in conjunction with these procedures is not mandatory and lacks scientific support. However, in cases of severe postoperative infection, extending beyond the surgical area, the administration of systemic antibiotics may be considered.

Another aspect that needs to be kept in mind when autogenous soft tissue grafts are used is the possibility of sensory changes that can occur after graft harvesting from the palate. Although the data are limited, the patients need to be informed on the possibility to have a transient or persistent numbness on the palatal surface following graft harvesting.[85,88]

Soft Tissue Replacement Materials

To overcome the drawbacks related to autogenous graft harvesting, alternative biomaterials, such as EMD, soft tissue replacement material, PRF, or HA, have been investigated.[35,89–91]

Xenogeneic and allogenic membranes as a substitute for CTG have been intensively tested in the past decade. Several clinical studies provided promising clinical results for root coverage when CTG substitutes, such as ADM,[91,92] EMD,[93,94] PRF,[95,96] or XCM,[32,33,38,97] have been used for the coverage of Miller class I, II, or III (RT1 and 2) GRs. Several studies have evaluated the effectiveness of various CTG substitutes associated to CAF for the treatment of RT1 (Miller class I and II) recession defects.[98] Based on results from 27 studies, the evaluated CTG substitutes (ADM, PRF, EMD, XCM) showed superior results compared with CAF alone. The network analyses indicated the treatment ranking of these substitutes, pointing to ADM as providing the best results, followed by PRF, EMD, and XCM.[98] However, when comparing CTG with ADM or XCM, another recent meta-analysis obtained comparable results in terms of relative root coverage (see **Fig. 3**).[99]

Enamel Matrix Derivative

Results from histologic animal and human studies have provided evidence that EMD induces periodontal regeneration (ie, formation of new cementum, new periodontal ligament, and bone) in the surgical treatment of GRs.[100–102] Several authors have reported improved results for root coverage in Miller class I and II recessions where EMD and CAF were used as compared with CAF alone.[61,103,104] A recent meta-analysis reported statistically significant better results for recession reduction and clinical attachment level (CAL) gain when EMD was associated to CAF or CAF + CTG.[105] In a recent clinical study evaluating the clinical results after 3 years, CTG + EMD provided significantly better outcomes for the percentage of mean root coverage (90.69% ± 10.10% for CTG + EMD, 79.25% ± 19.55% for CTG) and for residual recession depth (0.39 ± 0.19 mm for CTG + EMD, 0.92 ± 0.43 mm for CTG) compared with those treated with CTG alone.[106] Corroborating data were reported by Spahr and coworkers[107] pointing to better recession coverage and less recession recurrence after 2 years for the EMD group. Promising results were also reported when EMD was associated to CTG using MCAT for the treatment of single mandibular Miller class I and II recessions[72] or for maxillary MAGR.[94] However, the single use of EMD adjunctive to CAF seems to provide inferior clinical and aesthetic results as compared with

CTG + tunnel technique 5 years after surgery,[108] pointing to the fact that CTG remains the gold standard for achieving optimal recession coverage.

Platelet-Rich Fibrin

In the past years, PRF has been increasingly used for the surgical treatment of GRs.[95,109] Biologically, the concept is based on the slow and gradual release of growth factors from the fibrin-dense membrane obtained after blood centrifugation. Studies evaluating PRF adjunctive to CAF as opposed to CAF alone showed significantly better outcomes for root coverage and CAL gain favoring PRF.[96,110–112] This was also obtained in a recent meta-analysis, which pointed to statistically significant better outcomes for the relative recession coverage and CAL gain in cases where PRF was used.[34] When PRF was combined with CAF + CTG, statistically significantly better relative root coverage and CAL gain was obtained compared with CAF + CTG alone.[113] However, when CAF + PRF was compared with CTG, significantly better outcomes (root coverage, CAL gain, gain in keratinized gingiva) were obtained favoring the CTG group.[34,114]

Hyaluronic Acid

HA is a natural carbohydrate component of the extracellular matrix found in skin, joints, eyes, and periodontium and has hygroscopic, viscoelastic, anti-inflammatory, and antiedematous properties.[115–118] It also supports clot formation, angiogenesis, osteogenesis and cell adhesion, migration, and differentiation.[115,119,120] A recent histologic study in dogs has shown that the additional use of HA to CAF provides statistically significant better results for CAL, bone formation, formation of cementum, and connective tissue attachment compared with CAF alone.[36] Other reports confirm that adjunctive use of HA to CAF increases the probability of complete root coverage compared with CAF alone in Miller class I recessions.[115] Promising results were also obtained in single and multiple GRs treated with MCAT or the LCT and HA.[39,40] Nonetheless, further randomized clinical studies are needed to determine the adjunctive benefit of HA in the surgical treatment of GRs.

SUMMARY

Taken together, the use of a CTG with either CAF or tunnel seems to be the most predictable techniques for the treatment of single and multiple GRs. So far, long-term results (ie, 5-year follow-up or more) exist only for CAF with/without CTG providing evidence for long-term stability with only minor relapses. Soft tissue replacement materials and biologics may represent a valuable modality to additionally improve the clinical outcomes obtained with CAF alone or, in certain clinical situations, to serve as alternative to autogenous tissue.

CLINICS CARE POINTS

- Soft tissue healing after connective tissue graft or free gingival graft is characterised by a significant tissue shrinkage.
- The coronaly advanced flap is one of the best investigated surgical techniques for gingival recession coverage.
- The modified coronally advances tunnel (MCAT) has been develod in order to minimize the risks for flap perforation.
- The routine administration of antibiotics after surgical recession coverage procwdures lacks evidence and is not recommended.

- Alternative to autogenous grafts, biological materials such as an enamel matrix derivative, plasma rich fibrin, hyaluronic acid or sof tissue xenogeneic or allogenic replacement membranes have been investigated.

REFERENCES

1. Richmond S, Chestnutt I, Shennan J, et al. The relationship of medical and dental factors to perceived general and dental health. Community Dent Oral Epidemiol 2007;35:89–97.
2. Susin C, Haas AN, Oppermann RV, et al. Gingival recession: epidemiology and risk indicators in a representative urban Brazilian population. J Periodontol 2004;75:1377–86.
3. Thomson WM, Broadbent JM, Poulton R, et al. Changes in periodontal disease experience from 26 to 32 years of age in a birth cohort. J Periodontol 2006;77: 947–54.
4. Gorman WJ. Prevalence and etiology of gingival recession. J Periodontol 1967; 38:316–22.
5. Zucchelli G, Mounssif I. Periodontal plastic surgery. Periodontol 2000 2015;68: 333–68.
6. Loe H, Anerud A, Boysen H. The natural history of periodontal disease in man: prevalence, severity, and extent of gingival recession. J Periodontol 1992;63: 489–95.
7. Yoneyama T, Okamoto H, Lindhe J, et al. Probing depth, attachment loss and gingival recession. Findings from a clinical examination in Ushiku, Japan. J Clin Periodontol 1988;15:581–91.
8. Prato GP, Rotundo R, Magnani C, et al. Viral etiology of gingival recession. A case report. J Periodontol 2002;73:110–4.
9. Parma-Benfenali S, Fugazzoto PA, Ruben MP. The effect of restorative margins on the postsurgical development and nature of the periodontium. Part I. Int J Periodontics Restorative Dent 1985;5:30–51.
10. Stoner JE, Mazdyasna S. Gingival recession in the lower incisor region of 15-year-old subjects. J Periodontol 1980;51:74–6.
11. Camargo PM, Melnick PR, Kenney EB. The use of free gingival grafts for aesthetic purposes. Periodontol 2000 2001;27:72–96.
12. Chambrone L, Tatakis DN. Long-term outcomes of untreated buccal gingival recessions: a systematic review and meta-analysis. J Periodontol 2016;87:796–808.
13. Wennstrom JL, Lindhe J, Sinclair F, et al. Some periodontal tissue reactions to orthodontic tooth movement in monkeys. J Clin Periodontol 1987;14:121–9.
14. Cairo F. Periodontal plastic surgery of gingival recessions at single and multiple teeth. Periodontol 2000 2017;75:296–316.
15. Hathaway-Schrader JD, Novince CM. Maintaining homeostatic control of periodontal bone tissue. Periodontol 2000 2021;86:157–87.
16. Mombelli A. Maintenance therapy for teeth and implants. Periodontol 2000 2019;79:190–9.
17. Salzer S, Graetz C, Dorfer CE, et al. Contemporary practices for mechanical oral hygiene to prevent periodontal disease. Periodontol 2000 2020;84:35–44.
18. Baer PN, Benjamin SD. Gingival grafts: a historical note. J Periodontol 1981;52: 206–7.
19. Bernimoulin JP, Luscher B, Muhlemann HR. Coronally repositioned periodontal flap. Clinical evaluation after one year. J Clin Periodontol 1975;2:1–13.

20. Cohen DW, Ross SE. The double papillae repositioned flap in periodontal therapy. J Periodontol 1968;39:65–70.
21. Grupe HE. Modified technique for the sliding flap operation. J Periodontol 1966; 37:491–5.
22. Harris RJ. The connective tissue and partial thickness double pedicle graft: a predictable method of obtaining root coverage. J Periodontol 1992;63:477–86.
23. Harvey PM. Surgical reconstruction of the gingiva. II. Procedures. N Z Dent J 1970;66:42–52.
24. Langer B, Langer L. Subepithelial connective tissue graft technique for root coverage. J Periodontol 1985;56:715–20.
25. Nabers JM. Free gingival grafts. Periodontics 1966;4:243–5.
26. Sullivan HC, Atkins JH. Free autogenous gingival grafts. 3. Utilization of grafts in the treatment of gingival recession. Periodontics 1968;6:152–60.
27. Sumner CF 3rd. Surgical repair of recession on the maxillary cuspid: incisally repositioning the gingival tissues. J Periodontol 1969;40:119–21.
28. Cairo F, Cortellini P, Pilloni A, et al. Clinical efficacy of coronally advanced flap with or without connective tissue graft for the treatment of multiple adjacent gingival recessions in the aesthetic area: a randomized controlled clinical trial. J Clin Periodontol 2016;43:849–56.
29. Cairo F, Nieri M, Pagliaro U. Efficacy of periodontal plastic surgery procedures in the treatment of localized facial gingival recessions. A systematic review. J Clin Periodontol 2014;41(Suppl 15):S44–62.
30. Zucchelli G, Tavelli L, Barootchi S, et al. The influence of tooth location on the outcomes of multiple adjacent gingival recessions treated with coronally advanced flap: a multicenter re-analysis study. J Periodontol 2019;90:1244–51.
31. Aroca S, Keglevich T, Nikolidakis D, et al. Treatment of class III multiple gingival recessions: a randomized-clinical trial. J Clin Periodontol 2010;37:88–97.
32. Aroca S, Molnar B, Windisch P, et al. Treatment of multiple adjacent Miller class I and II gingival recessions with a modified coronally advanced tunnel (MCAT) technique and a collagen matrix or palatal connective tissue graft: a randomized, controlled clinical trial. J Clin Periodontol 2013;40:713–20.
33. Cosgarea R, Juncar R, Arweiler N, et al. Clinical evaluation of a porcine acellular dermal matrix for the treatment of multiple adjacent class I, II, and III gingival recessions using the modified coronally advanced tunnel technique. Quintessence Int 2016;47:739–47.
34. Miron RJ, Moraschini V, Del Fabbro M, et al. Use of platelet-rich fibrin for the treatment of gingival recessions: a systematic review and meta-analysis. Clin Oral Investig 2020;24:2543–57.
35. Roccuzzo M, Lungo M, Corrente G, et al. Comparative study of a bioresorbable and a non-resorbable membrane in the treatment of human buccal gingival recessions. J Periodontol 1996;67:7–14.
36. Shirakata Y, Nakamura T, Kawakami Y, et al. Healing of buccal gingival recessions following treatment with coronally advanced flap alone or combined with a cross-linked hyaluronic acid gel. An experimental study in dogs. J Clin Periodontol 2021;48:570–80.
37. Woodyard JG, Greenwell H, Hill M, et al. The clinical effect of acellular dermal matrix on gingival thickness and root coverage compared to coronally positioned flap alone. J Periodontol 2004;75:44–56.
38. Cosgarea R, Miron R, Bora R, et al. Long-term results after treatment of multiple adjacent gingival recessions with the modified coronally advanced tunnel and a porcine acellular dermal matrix. Quintessence Int 2021;52:32–44.

39. Lanzrein C, Guldener K, Imber JC, et al. Treatment of multiple adjacent recessions with the modified coronally advanced tunnel or laterally closed tunnel in conjunction with cross-linked hyaluronic acid and subepithelial connective tissue graft: a report of 15 cases. Quintessence Int 2020;51:710–9.
40. Guldener K, Lanzrein C, Eliezer M, et al. Treatment of single mandibular recessions with the modified coronally advanced tunnel or laterally closed tunnel, hyaluronic acid, and subepithelial connective tissue graft: a report of 12 cases. Quintessence Int 2020;51:456–63.
41. Caffesse RG, Burgett FG, Nasjleti CE, et al. Healing of free gingival grafts with and without periosteum. Part I. Histologic evaluation. J Periodontol 1979;50: 586–94.
42. Caffesse RG, Nasjleti CE, Castelli WA. The role of sulcular environment in controlling epithelial keratinization. J Periodontol 1979;50:1–6.
43. Egli U, Vollmer WH, Rateitschak KH. Follow-up studies of free gingival grafts. J Clin Periodontol 1975;2:98–104.
44. James WC, McFall WT Jr. Placement of free gingival grafts on denuded alveolar bone. Part I: clinical evaluations. J Periodontol 1978;49:283–90.
45. Mormann W, Schaer F, Firestone AR. The relationship between success of free gingival grafts and transplant thickness. Revascularization and shrinkage: a one year clinical study. J Periodontol 1981;52:74–80.
46. Oliver RC, Loe H, Karring T. Microscopic evaluation of the healing and revascularization of free gingival grafts. J Periodontal Res 1968;3:84–95.
47. Orsini M, Orsini G, Benlloch D, et al. Esthetic and dimensional evaluation of free connective tissue grafts in prosthetically treated patients: a 1-year clinical study. J Periodontol 2004;75:470–7.
48. Staffileno H Jr, Levy S. Histologic and clinical study of mucosal (gingival) transplants in dogs. J Periodontol 1969;40:311–9.
49. Rateitschak KH, Egli U, Fringeli G. Recession: a 4-year longitudinal study after free gingival grafts. J Clin Periodontol 1979;6:158–64.
50. Karring T, Ostergaard E, Loe H. Conservation of tissue specificity after heterotopic transplantation of gingiva and alveolar mucosa. J Periodontal Res 1971; 6:282–93.
51. Wennstrom J. Regeneration of gingiva following surgical excision. A clinical study. J Clin Periodontol 1983;10:287–97.
52. Wennstrom J, Lindhe J. Role of attached gingiva for maintenance of periodontal health. Healing following excisional and grafting procedures in dogs. J Clin Periodontol 1983;10:206–21.
53. Wennstrom J, Lindhe J, Nyman S. Role of keratinized gingiva for gingival health. Clinical and histologic study of normal and regenerated gingival tissue in dogs. J Clin Periodontol 1981;8:311–28.
54. Karring T, Lang NP, Loe H. The role of gingival connective tissue in determining epithelial differentiation. J Periodontal Res 1975;10:1–11.
55. Edel A. Clinical evaluation of free connective tissue grafts used to increase the width of keratinised gingiva. J Clin Periodontol 1974;1:185–96.
56. Edel A, Faccini JM. Histologic changes following the grafting of connective tissue into human gingiva. Oral Surg Oral Med Oral Pathol 1977;43:190–5.
57. Ouhayoun JP, Sawaf MH, Gofflaux JC, et al. Re-epithelialization of a palatal connective tissue graft transplanted in a non-keratinized alveolar mucosa: a histological and biochemical study in humans. J Periodontal Res 1988;23:127–33.
58. Bernimoulin JP, Lange DE. [Effects of heterotopic connective tissue transplantation on epithelium regeneration]. Dtsch Zahnarztl Z 1973;28:202–5.

59. Bernimoulin JP, Schroeder HE. Changes in the differentiation pattern of oral mucosal epithelium following heterotopic connective tissue transplantation in man. Pathol Res Pract 1980;166:290–312.

60. Lange DE, Bernimoulin JP. Exfoliative cytological studies in evaluation of free gingival graft healing. J Clin Periodontol 1974;1:89–96.

61. Cairo F, Pagliaro U, Nieri M. Treatment of gingival recession with coronally advanced flap procedures: a systematic review. J Clin Periodontol 2008;35:136–62.

62. Cairo F, Rotundo R, Miller PD, et al. Root coverage esthetic score: a system to evaluate the esthetic outcome of the treatment of gingival recession through evaluation of clinical cases. J Periodontol 2009;80:705–10.

63. Hofmanner P, Alessandri R, Laugisch O, et al. Predictability of surgical techniques used for coverage of multiple adjacent gingival recessions: a systematic review. Quintessence Int 2012;43:545–54.

64. Prato GP, Clauser C, Cortellini P. Periodontal plastic and mucogingival surgery. Periodontol 2000 1995;9:90–105.

65. Cortellini P, Tonetti M, Prato GP. The partly epithelialized free gingival graft (PE-FGG) at lower incisors. A pilot study with implications for alignment of the mucogingival junction. J Clin Periodontol 2012;39:674–80.

66. da Silva RC, Joly JC, de Lima AF, et al. Root coverage using the coronally positioned flap with or without a subepithelial connective tissue graft. J Periodontol 2004;75:413–9.

67. Pini Prato G, Rotundo R, Franceschi D, et al. Fourteen-year outcomes of coronally advanced flap for root coverage: follow-up from a randomized trial. J Clin Periodontol 2011;38:715–20.

68. Zucchelli G, De Sanctis M. Long-term outcome following treatment of multiple Miller class I and II recession defects in esthetic areas of the mouth. J Periodontol 2005;76:2286–92.

69. de Sanctis M, Zucchelli G. Coronally advanced flap: a modified surgical approach for isolated recession-type defects: three-year results. J Clin Periodontol 2007;34:262–8.

70. Stimmelmayr M, Allen EP, Gernet W, et al. Treatment of gingival recession in the anterior mandible using the tunnel technique and a combination epithelialized-subepithelial connective tissue graft-a case series. Int J Periodontics Restorative Dent 2011;31:165–73.

71. Sculean A, Allen EP. The laterally closed tunnel for the treatment of deep isolated mandibular recessions: surgical technique and a report of 24 cases. Int J Periodontics Restorative Dent 2018;38:479–87.

72. Sculean A, Cosgarea R, Stahli A, et al. The modified coronally advanced tunnel combined with an enamel matrix derivative and subepithelial connective tissue graft for the treatment of isolated mandibular Miller class I and II gingival recessions: a report of 16 cases. Quintessence Int 2014;45:829–35.

73. Graziani F, Gennai S, Roldan S, et al. Efficacy of periodontal plastic procedures in the treatment of multiple gingival recessions. J Clin Periodontol 2014;41(Suppl 15):S63–76.

74. Zucchelli G, De Sanctis M. Treatment of multiple recession-type defects in patients with esthetic demands. J Periodontol 2000;71:1506–14.

75. Bertl K, Spineli LM, Mohandis K, et al. Root coverage stability: a systematic overview of controlled clinical trials with at least 5 years of follow-up. Clin Exp Dent Res 2021;1–19.

76. Chambrone L, Ortega MAS, Sukekava F, et al. Root coverage procedures for treating single and multiple recession-type defects: an updated Cochrane systematic review. J Periodontol 2019;90:1399–422.

77. Zuhr O, Rebele SF, Cheung SL, et al. Research Group on Oral Soft Tissue B, Wound H. Surgery without papilla incision: tunneling flap procedures in plastic periodontal and implant surgery. Periodontol 2000 2018;77:123–49.

78. Cosgarea R, Arweiler N, Sculean A. Die Behandlung von singulären und multiplen Rezessionen mit der modifizierten Tunneltechnik. Dent Implantol 2013;17: 256–64.

79. Buti J, Baccini M, Nieri M, et al. Bayesian network meta-analysis of root coverage procedures: ranking efficacy and identification of best treatment. J Clin Periodontol 2013;40:372–86.

80. Zucchelli G, Marzadori M, Mounssif I, et al. Coronally advanced flap + connective tissue graft techniques for the treatment of deep gingival recession in the lower incisors. A controlled randomized clinical trial. J Clin Periodontol 2014; 41:806–13.

81. Pini-Prato GP, Cairo F, Nieri M, et al. Coronally advanced flap versus connective tissue graft in the treatment of multiple gingival recessions: a split-mouth study with a 5-year follow-up. J Clin Periodontol 2010;37:644–50.

82. Dai A, Huang JP, Ding PH, et al. Long-term stability of root coverage procedures for single gingival recessions: a systematic review and meta-analysis. J Clin Periodontol 2019;46:572–85.

83. Rasperini G, Acunzo R, Pellegrini G, et al. Predictor factors for long-term outcomes stability of coronally advanced flap with or without connective tissue graft in the treatment of single maxillary gingival recessions: 9 years results of a randomized controlled clinical trial. J Clin Periodontol 2018;45:1107–17.

84. Cairo F, Cortellini P, Tonetti M, et al. Stability of root coverage outcomes at single maxillary gingival recession with loss of interdental attachment: 3-year extension results from a randomized, controlled, clinical trial. J Clin Periodontol 2015;42: 575–81.

85. Chackartchi T, Romanos GE, Sculean A. Soft tissue-related complications and management around dental implants. Periodontol 2000 2019;81:124–38.

86. Fu JH, Hasso DG, Yeh CY, et al. The accuracy of identifying the greater palatine neurovascular bundle: a cadaver study. J Periodontol 2011;82:1000–6.

87. Reiser GM, Bruno JF, Mahan PE, et al. The subepithelial connective tissue graft palatal donor site: anatomic considerations for surgeons. Int J Periodontics Restorative Dent 1996;16:130–7.

88. Buff LR, Burklin T, Eickholz P, et al. Does harvesting connective tissue grafts from the palate cause persistent sensory dysfunction? A pilot study. Quintessence Int 2009;40:479–89.

89. Barker TS, Cueva MA, Rivera-Hidalgo F, et al. A comparative study of root coverage using two different acellular dermal matrix products. J Periodontol 2010;81:1596–603.

90. Zucchelli G, Clauser C, De Sanctis M, et al. Mucogingival versus guided tissue regeneration procedures in the treatment of deep recession type defects. J Periodontol 1998;69:138–45.

91. McGuire MK, Scheyer ET. Randomized, controlled clinical trial to evaluate a xenogeneic collagen matrix as an alternative to free gingival grafting for oral soft tissue augmentation. J Periodontol 2014;85:1333–41.

92. Reis MBL, Mandetta CMR, Dantas CDF, et al. Root coverage of gingival recessions with non-carious cervical lesions: a controlled clinical trial. Clin Oral Investig 2020;24:4583–9.

93. Sangiorgio JPM, Neves F, Rocha Dos Santos M, et al. Xenogenous collagen matrix and/or enamel matrix derivative for treatment of localized gingival recessions: a randomized clinical trial. Part I: clinical outcomes. J Periodontol 2017; 88:1309–18.

94. Sculean A, Cosgarea R, Stahli A, et al. Treatment of multiple adjacent maxillary Miller class I, II, and III gingival recessions with the modified coronally advanced tunnel, enamel matrix derivative, and subepithelial connective tissue graft: a report of 12 cases. Quintessence Int 2016;47:653–9.

95. Moraschini V, Barboza Edos S. Use of platelet-rich fibrin membrane in the treatment of gingival recession: a systematic review and meta-analysis. J Periodontol 2016;87:281–90.

96. Aroca S, Keglevich T, Barbieri B, et al. Clinical evaluation of a modified coronally advanced flap alone or in combination with a platelet-rich fibrin membrane for the treatment of adjacent multiple gingival recessions: a 6-month study. J Periodontol 2009;80:244–52.

97. Molnar B, Aroca S, Keglevich T, et al. Treatment of multiple adjacent Miller class I and II gingival recessions with collagen matrix and the modified coronally advanced tunnel technique. Quintessence Int 2013;44:17–24.

98. Moraschini V, Calasans-Maia MD, Dias AT, et al. Effectiveness of connective tissue graft substitutes for the treatment of gingival recessions compared with coronally advanced flap: a network meta-analysis. Clin Oral Investig 2020;24: 3395–406.

99. de Carvalho Formiga M, Nagasawa MA, Moraschini V, et al. Clinical efficacy of xenogeneic and allogeneic 3D matrix in the management of gingival recession: a systematic review and meta-analysis. Clin Oral Investig 2020;24:2229–45.

100. McGuire MK, Cochran DL. Evaluation of human recession defects treated with coronally advanced flaps and either enamel matrix derivative or connective tissue. Part 2: Histological evaluation. J Periodontol 2003;74:1126–35.

101. Franca-Grohmann IL, Sangiorgio JPM, Bueno MR, et al. Treatment of dehiscence-type defects with collagen matrix and/or enamel matrix derivative: histomorphometric study in minipigs. J Periodontol 2020;91:967–74.

102. McGuire MK, Scheyer ET, Schupbach P. A prospective, case-controlled study evaluating the use of enamel matrix derivative on human buccal recession defects: a human histologic examination. J Periodontol 2016;87:645–53.

103. Koop R, Merheb J, Quirynen M. Periodontal regeneration with enamel matrix derivative in reconstructive periodontal therapy: a systematic review. J Periodontol 2012;83:707–20.

104. Chambrone L, Pannuti CM, Tu YK, et al. Evidence-based periodontal plastic surgery. II. An individual data meta-analysis for evaluating factors in achieving complete root coverage. J Periodontol 2012;83:477–90.

105. Meza Mauricio J, Furquim CP, Bustillos-Torrez W, et al. Does enamel matrix derivative application provide additional clinical benefits in the treatment of maxillary Miller class I and II gingival recession? A systematic review and meta-analysis. Clin Oral Investig 2021;25:1613–26.

106. Mercado F, Hamlet S, Ivanovski S. A 3-year prospective clinical and patient-centered trial on subepithelial connective tissue graft with or without enamel matrix derivative in class I-II Miller recessions. J Periodontal Res 2020;55:296–306.

107. Spahr A, Haegewald S, Tsoulfidou F, et al. Coverage of Miller class I and II recession defects using enamel matrix proteins versus coronally advanced flap technique: a 2-year report. J Periodontol 2005;76:1871–80.
108. Zuhr O, Akakpo D, Eickholz P, et al. Tunnel technique with connective tissue graft versus coronally advanced flap with enamel matrix derivate for root coverage: 5-year results of an RCT using 3D digital measurement technology for volumetric comparison of soft tissue changes. J Clin Periodontol 2021;48: 949–61.
109. Miron RJ, Zucchelli G, Pikos MA, et al. Use of platelet-rich fibrin in regenerative dentistry: a systematic review. Clin Oral Investig 2017;21:1913–27.
110. Padma R, Shilpa A, Kumar PA, et al. A split mouth randomized controlled study to evaluate the adjunctive effect of platelet-rich fibrin to coronally advanced flap in Miller's class-I and II recession defects. J Indian Soc Periodontol 2013;17: 631–6.
111. Kuka S, Ipci SD, Cakar G, et al. Clinical evaluation of coronally advanced flap with or without platelet-rich fibrin for the treatment of multiple gingival recessions. Clin Oral Investig 2018;22:1551–8.
112. Bozkurt Dogan S, Ongoz Dede F, Balli U, et al. Concentrated growth factor in the treatment of adjacent multiple gingival recessions: a split-mouth randomized clinical trial. J Clin Periodontol 2015;42:868–75.
113. Keceli HG, Kamak G, Erdemir EO, et al. The adjunctive effect of platelet-rich fibrin to connective tissue graft in the treatment of buccal recession defects: results of a randomized, parallel-group controlled trial. J Periodontol 2015;86: 1221–30.
114. Jankovic S, Aleksic Z, Klokkevold P, et al. Use of platelet-rich fibrin membrane following treatment of gingival recession: a randomized clinical trial. Int J Periodontics Restorative Dent 2012;32:e41–50.
115. Pilloni A, Schmidlin PR, Sahrmann P, et al. Effectiveness of adjunctive hyaluronic acid application in coronally advanced flap in Miller class I single gingival recession sites: a randomized controlled clinical trial. Clin Oral Investig 2019;23: 1133–41.
116. Eliezer M, Imber JC, Sculean A, et al. Hyaluronic acid as adjunctive to non-surgical and surgical periodontal therapy: a systematic review and meta-analysis. Clin Oral Investig 2019;23:3423–35.
117. de Brito Bezerra B, Mendes Brazao MA, de Campos ML, et al. Association of hyaluronic acid with a collagen scaffold may improve bone healing in critical-size bone defects. Clin Oral Implants Res 2012;23:938–42.
118. Dahiya P, Kamal R. Hyaluronic acid: a boon in periodontal therapy. N Am J Med Sci 2013;5:309–15.
119. Asparuhova MB, Chappuis V, Stahli A, et al. Role of hyaluronan in regulating self-renewal and osteogenic differentiation of mesenchymal stromal cells and pre-osteoblasts. Clin Oral Investig 2020;24:3923–37.
120. Oksala O, Salo T, Tammi R, et al. Expression of proteoglycans and hyaluronan during wound healing. J Histochem Cytochem 1995;43:125–35.

Regenerative Periodontal Therapy in Intrabony Defects and Long-Term Tooth Prognosis

Andreas Stavropoulos, DDS, PhD, Dr. Odont.[a,b,*],
Kristina Bertl, DDS, MSc, MBA, PhD[a,c], Anton Sculean, DMD, MS, PhD[d],
Alpdogan Kantarci, DDS, PhD[e]

KEYWORDS

- Periodontal regeneration • Bone grafts • Bone substitutes • GTR
- Enamel matrix proteins • EMD • Long term

KEY POINTS

- Periodontal regenerative procedures yield significantly better clinical outcomes in intrabony defects compared with open flap debridement, on the medium- to long-term.
- Combination approaches, including the use of a bone graft seem to be more efficacious compared with monotherapy.
- Periodontal regenerative procedures result in higher rates of tooth preservation compared with open flap debridement on the medium- to long-term.

WHY PERIODONTAL REGENERATIVE PROCEDURES?

To arrest progressive attachment loss and/or prevent further disease progression, control of the infection caused by the oral bacterial biofilm remains the primary aim of periodontal treatment. For most patients and teeth/sites, this goal can be commonly achieved through proper and adequate self-performed oral hygiene and professionally performed nonsurgical and/or conventional surgical periodontal treatment. In the clinic, this translates into reduced probing pocket depths (PD) and gain in clinical attachment level (CAL), reduced tendency to bleeding on probing (BoP), and stable/increased bone

[a] Department of Periodontology, Faculty of Odontology, University of Malmö, Carl Gustafs väg 34, SE- 20506, Malmö 214 21, Sweden; [b] Division of Conservative Dentistry and Periodontology, University Clinic of Dentistry, Medical University of Vienna, Sensengasse 2, AT-1090 Wien, Austria; [c] Division of Oral Surgery, University Clinic of Dentistry, Medical University of Vienna, Sensengasse 2, AT-1090 Wien, Austria; [d] Department of Periodontology, School of Dental Medicine, University of Bern, Freiburgstrasse 7, 3010 Bern, Switzerland; [e] Forsyth Institute, 245 First Street, Cambridge, MA 02142, USA
* Corresponding author. Department of Periodontology, Faculty of Odontology, University of Malmö, Sweden.
E-mail address: andreas.stavropoulos@mau.se

Dent Clin N Am 66 (2022) 103–109
https://doi.org/10.1016/j.cden.2021.09.002
0011-8532/22/© 2021 The Authors. Published by Elsevier Inc. This is an open access article under the CC BY-NC-ND license (http://creativecommons.org/licenses/by-nc-nd/4.0/).
dental.theclinics.com

levels, compared with pretreatment levels. Nevertheless, residual (deep) PD can still be present following nonsurgical and/or conventional surgical periodontal therapy, commonly in teeth/sites with deep intrabony defects and/or deep furcation involvements. Deep PD after periodontal therapy is indeed associated with an increased risk for disease progression and tooth loss. In a long-term study,[1] deep residual PD or a deep furcation involvement (ie, class II and III) after treatment has been associated with an exponential higher risk for periodontitis progression and tooth loss. Specifically, a greater than 10 times higher risk for tooth loss has been reported for teeth with a residual PD greater than or equal to 6 mm compared with teeth with a residual PD of less than or equal to 3 mm, whereas teeth with a class II or III furcation involvement showed about 5 to 13 times higher risk for tooth loss compared with teeth with no furcation involvement.[1] Deep defects can be managed efficiently with either resective or regenerative approaches. Resective approaches, however, have the drawback of extensive soft tissue recession and often further loss of attachment.[2-4] Thus, a variety of surgical regenerative treatment protocols have been developed and refined during the last 3 to 4 decades, with the aim to enhance treatment outcomes and at the same time to evade/reduce the aforementioned shortcomings of conventional and/or resective approaches. Indeed, significantly better clinical (ie, larger CAL gains, shallower residual PD, and less recession) and radiographic results (ie, larger bone level gain and reduced residual intrabony defects) have been collectively reported after regenerative periodontal procedures compared with conventional surgical procedures. Periodontal regenerative procedures—as the term coins—result also in significantly better histologic outcomes compared with conventional surgery (ie, larger amounts of new cementum, periodontal ligament, and alveolar bone) if correct case selection, appropriate execution of treatment, and undisturbed healing are provided (for review see[5,6]).

LONGEVITY OF TREATMENT

The overall goal of periodontal therapy is to reestablish periodontal health and contribute to the overall oral well-being, that is, having only a few sites with bleeding on probing and no teeth with deep PD, the teeth are capable of functioning trouble-free, and preferably there is a satisfactory esthetic appearance. This goal should be achieved by preserving as many teeth as possible, for as long as possible. It is well established that the clinical conditions obtained after conventional periodontal therapy, nonsurgical or surgical, can be maintained for several decades, provided that the patient is keeping an adequate oral hygiene level.[7,8] Thus, if one treatment should be considered better than conventional periodontal therapy, the results of this treatment should also be maintainable for a long period. In this context, the histologic outcomes obtained after periodontal regenerative procedures show variability in terms of the relative tissue composition of the various constituents of the periodontium, mainly depending on the use and/or the type of biomaterial and/or bone substitute.[6,9] For example, the use of deproteinized bovine bone—a barely resorbable material—results in a regenerated periodontium, where the new bone tissue contains a substantial number of the grafted particles after completed healing[10,11] (**Fig. 1**). It is thus relevant to assess the long-term outcome of the various periodontal regenerative procedures and the possible impact of presence of graft substitute particles within the tissues. In the following section, results from a relatively recently performed systematic appraisal of the literature on the long-term outcome of regenerative periodontal treatment in intrabony defects are shortly discussed.[12] In the recent systematic literature search, only publications from randomized clinical trials on regenerative periodontal treatment with an average follow-up greater than or equal to 3 years, but with a

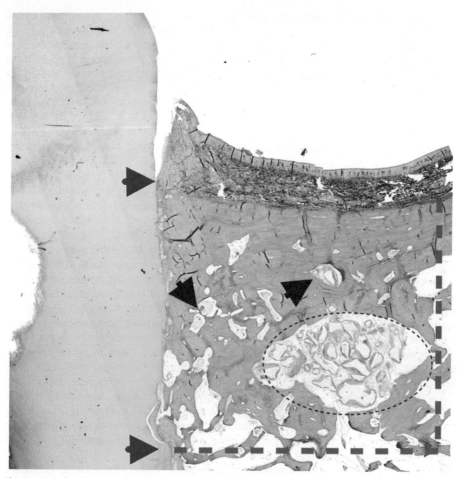

Fig. 1. Histologic image from the molar of a dog, where a large box-type defect (outlined by the dotted *green line*) was grafted with a deproteinized bovine bone/collagen construct and covered with a collagen membrane, 1.5 years after treatment. Complete regeneration of the periodontium was observed (*red arrows* indicate the bottom of the original defect and the coronal extension of new cementum formation), whereas graft particles (*blue arrowheads*) could be observed completely engulfed within the new bone. Occasionally, large numbers of particles were aggregated in dense connective tissue within bone cavities (outlined by the *dotted blue line*).

minimum follow-up greater than or equal to 2 years, were identified, which is already setting the bar high for the decision-making for the success of regenerative procedures. In perspective, what is appropriate longevity of treatment may be a matter of debate, and aspects of professional effort and cost-effectiveness, as well as patient-related outcomes including suffering should be taken into account. However, the success of any treatment modality should be tested and established over time.

LONG-TERM OUTCOMES IN INTRABONY DEFECTS

Thirty publications from a medium timeframe of 3 to 5 years (19 studies) and long-term of greater than 5 years (11 studies) were identified up to 04/2020, reporting on the following 6 regenerative/reconstructive approaches: (1) grafting, (2) guided tissue regeneration (GTR), (3) enamel matrix derivatives (EMD), (4) GTR + grafting, (5) EMD + grafting, and (6) various combinations, including those using different type of blood-derived growth factor constructs (BC). The treatments mostly reported on were GTR and EMD, without any adjunct use of a bone graft/substitute (14 and 9 different groups, respectively), and GTR was mostly performed with resorbable membranes (only 5 groups out of 24 used nonresorbable membranes). The most used grafting materials were alloplasts (11 groups) and xenografts (8 groups), whereas 5 groups combined BC with GTR, EMD, and/or bone grafts. Nine studies provided information on the long-term outcome of conventional periodontal surgery (ie, open flap debridement [OFD]).

On average, residual PD ranged from 3.9 ± 1.5 mm to 5.6 ± 1.1 mm and from 4.5 ± 1.8 mm to 7.6 ± 2.1 mm at the medium and long term, respectively, in teeth treated with OFD. The corresponding values from teeth treated with a regenerative approach ranged from 2.1 ± 0.4 mm (in a group treated with EMD + BC) to 4.7 ± 1.2 mm (in a group treated with GTR) at the medium term and from 2.9 ± 0.9 mm to 5.8 ± 1.9 mm (both in GTR groups) in the long term. Collectively, residual PD after regenerative/reconstructive approaches was on average at a level that is considered maintainable by regular maintenance treatment, that is, less than 5 mm, in most of the included groups (47 out of 50 groups reporting on residual PD; 94%), whereas this was the case in only 4 out of 9 groups treated with OFD (**Fig. 2**). As mentioned earlier, presence of deep pockets greater than or equal to 6 mm showed a greater than 10 times higher risk for tooth loss compared with teeth with no pockets.[1]

In regard with CAL, the range was 0.8 ± 1.4 mm to 1.7 ± 1.3 mm and -1.2 ± 2.4 mm to 3.7 ± 3.4 mm at the medium and long term, respectively, in teeth treated with OFD. The corresponding values in teeth treated with a regenerative approach ranged from 1.6 ± 1.5 (GTR) mm to 5.4 ± 1.2 mm (grafting + BC) at the medium term and from 1.5 ± 1.2 mm to 5.2 ± 2.6 mm (both in GTR groups) in the long term. Collectively, CAL gain after regenerative/reconstructive approaches was on average greater than or equal to 3 mm in more than half of the groups (29 out of 54 groups; 54%), whereas this was the case in only 1 out of 9 groups treated with OFD.

Furthermore, by means of a network meta-analysis, it was attempted to provide a hierarchy of treatment, that is, which treatment was superior in terms of residual PD and CAL gain. The more efficacious treatments were found to be combination approaches including the use of a bone graft/substitute (eg, GTR + grafting, EMD + grafting), which means that monotherapies presented with relatively deeper residual PD and less CAL gain, compared with combination approaches. Indeed, in recent systematic reviews of preclinical[13] and human histologic studies[6] on regenerative periodontal therapy, sole implantation of bone grafts and/or substitutes in periodontal defects does not predictably lead to substantial amounts of periodontal regeneration. Rather, a portion of the bone graft/substitute particles often remains encapsulated within connective tissue. In contrast, grafting in combination with another regenerative approach (eg, GTR or EMD) gives larger and more predictable outcomes. In this context, it must be mentioned that grafting, in combination with a BC, does not necessarily enhance the outcome of treatment significantly compared with only grafting. Specifically, as reported in other recent systematic reviews, use of platelet-rich plasma[14] or platelet-derived growth factor[15] failed to provide any significant additional benefit in terms of clinical results, whereas use of platelet-rich fibrin (PRF) seems to result in significantly better clinical improvements compared with only grafting.[16] Nevertheless, there is scarce information regarding the medium- or long-term outcome of treatment with adjunct use of PRF.

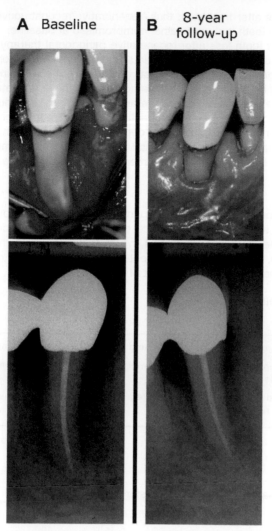

A Baseline   **B** 8-year follow-up

Fig. 2. (*A*).Pre-operative radiograph and intra-surgical photograph of a tooth harboring deep intrabony defect at its mesial and distal aspect, which was treated with EMD, as mono-therapy. (*B*) Radiograph and clinical photograph of the tooth 8, years post-operatively.

LONG-TERM TOOTH SURVIVAL

As discussed earlier, periodontal treatment aims to preserve as many teeth as possible, for as long as possible. Among the studies included in the aforementioned review,[12] 25 publications reported on tooth loss. In general, tooth loss was scarce, with only a fraction of studies reporting loss of greater than or equal to 1 tooth; specifically, only 0.4% of the teeth treated with a regenerative/reconstructive approach were lost due to recurrent periodontitis, whereas the corresponding number of lost teeth, previously treated with OFD, was 2.8%. Thus, the better clinical improvements observed after regenerative/reconstructive treatment on the medium to long term can be translated into increased tooth retention/survival. Importantly, most teeth were lost only from 5 years after treatment; thus, regenerative/reconstructive treatment supported survival of teeth that were rather compromised at baseline.

The low rate of tooth loss after regenerative periodontal therapy is related to the observation that only a fraction of the treated teeth experienced some limited extent loss of the CAL gain obtained postoperatively. Further, these findings imply that the mere presence of bone graft/substitute particles within the regenerated/reconstructed periodontal tissues does not have per se any negative consequence on periodontal homeostasis over the years. In perspective, disease recurrence and tooth loss following periodontal therapy are largely dependent on patient compliance, including maintenance therapy and/or general dental care,[7,8,17] as well as smoking habits, and should not solely be attributed to a treatment delivered several years earlier.

SUMMARY

Periodontal regenerative procedures, in particular combination approaches including grafting, result in significantly better clinical outcomes in intrabony defects, compared with OFD, on a medium to long term. This, in turn, translates into higher tooth retention in the long term, and therefore, periodontal regenerative/reconstructive therapy is strongly recommended for the treatment of intrabony defects.

CLINICS CARE POINTS

- Periodontal regeneration is a predictable and successful treatment for intrabony defects.
- Successful regeneration of periodontal defects will enable the clinicians and patients to retain natural teeth.
- Compliance and elimination of risk factors (eg. smoking) are critical for the long-term success of periodontal regenerative procedures.

DISCLOSURE

The authors declare no conflict of interest in regard with the present work.

REFERENCES

1. Matuliene G, Pjetursson BE, Salvi GE, et al. Influence of residual pockets on progression of periodontitis and tooth loss: results after 11 years of maintenance. J Clin Periodontol 2008;35:685–95.
2. Badersten A, Nilvéus R, Egelberg J. Scores of plaque, bleeding, suppuration and probing depth to predict probing attachment loss. 5 years of observation following nonsurgical periodontal therapy. J Clin Periodontol 1990;17:102–7.
3. Claffey N, Nylund K, Kiger R, et al. Diagnostic predictability of scores of plaque, bleeding, suppuration and probing depth for probing attachment loss. 3 1/2 years of observation following initial periodontal therapy. J Clin Periodontol 1990;17:108–14.
4. Kaldahl WB, Kalkwarf KL, Patil KD, et al. Long-term evaluation of periodontal therapy: I. Response to 4 therapeutic modalities. J Periodontol 1996;67:93–102.
5. Kao RT, Nares S, Reynolds MA. Periodontal regeneration - intrabony defects: a systematic review from the AAP Regeneration Workshop. J Periodontol 2015; 86:S77–104.

6. Sculean A, Nikolidakis D, Nikou G, et al. Biomaterials for promoting periodontal regeneration in human intrabony defects: a systematic review. Periodontol 2000 2015;68:182–216.
7. Axelsson P, Nyström B, Lindhe J. The long-term effect of a plaque control program on tooth mortality, caries and periodontal disease in adults. Results after 30 years of maintenance. J Clin Periodontol 2004;31:749–57.
8. Matuliene G, Studer R, Lang NP, et al. Significance of Periodontal Risk Assessment in the recurrence of periodontitis and tooth loss. J Clin Periodontol 2010; 37:191–9.
9. Laugisch O, Cosgarea R, Nikou G, et al. Histologic evidence of periodontal regeneration in furcation defects: a systematic review. Clin Oral Investig 2019; 23:2861–906.
10. Sculean AC, Arweiler N, Becker J, et al. Five-year clinical and histologic results following treatment of human intrabony defects with an enamel matrix derivative combined with a natural bone mineral. Int J Periodontics Restorative Dent 2008; 28:8.
11. Stavropoulos A, Wikesjö UM. Influence of defect dimensions on periodontal wound healing/regeneration in intrabony defects following implantation of a bovine bone biomaterial and provisions for guided tissue regeneration: an experimental study in the dog. J Clin Periodontol 2010;37:534–43.
12. Stavropoulos A, Bertl K, Spineli LM, et al. Medium- and long-term clinical benefits of periodontal regenerative/reconstructive procedures in intrabony defects: Systematic review and network meta-analysis of randomized controlled clinical studies. J Clin Periodontol 2021;48:410–30.
13. Ivanovic A, Nikou G, Miron RJ, et al. Which biomaterials may promote periodontal regeneration in intrabony periodontal defects? A systematic review of preclinical studies. Quintessence Int 2014;45:385–95.
14. Hou X, Yuan J, Aisaiti A, et al. The effect of platelet-rich plasma on clinical outcomes of the surgical treatment of periodontal intrabony defects: a systematic review and meta-analysis. BMC Oral Health 2016;16:71.
15. Khoshkam V, Chan HL, Lin GH, et al. Outcomes of regenerative treatment with rhPDGF-BB and rhFGF-2 for periodontal intra-bony defects: a systematic review and meta-analysis. J Clin Periodontol 2015;42:272–80.
16. Miron RJ, Moraschini V, Fujioka-Kobayashi M, et al. Use of platelet-rich fibrin for the treatment of periodontal intrabony defects: a systematic review and meta-analysis. Clin Oral Investig 2021;25(5):2461–78.
17. Löe H, Anerud A, Boysen H, et al. The natural history of periodontal disease in man. Tooth mortality rates before 40 years of age. J Periodontal Res 1978;13: 563–72.

Scaffolds in Periodontal Regenerative Treatment

Shuntaro Yamada, DDS, MSc[a], Siddharth Shanbhag, DDS, PhD[a,b],
Kamal Mustafa, DDS, PhD[a,*]

KEYWORDS

- Periodontal regeneration • Biomimetic • scaffolds • 3D printing • Tissue engineering

KEY POINTS

- Periodontal regeneration requires the hierarchical reorganization of soft and hard tissues, namely, periodontal ligament, cementum, alveolar bone, and gingiva.
- Three-dimensional microporous scaffolds offer structural support and spatiotemporal guidance for cell growth and differentiation.
- Biomimetic periodontal extracellular matrix scaffold may be produced by combining periodontal ligament cells and microporous scaffolds with the prospect of off-the-shelf products.
- Selection of scaffold architecture, functionalization techniques, and cell types determines the functionality of scaffolds.
- Three-dimensional printing technology allows for designing personalized scaffolds for periodontal regeneration.

INTRODUCTION

Advanced periodontitis results in the damage and loss of hard and soft tissues, which impairs oral function, aesthetics, and the patient's overall quality of life.[1] Although conventional therapies such as scaling and root plaining and flap surgery effectively interrupt disease progression, it often necessitates regenerative interventions to regain the original architecture and function of periodontal tissues because of limitation in spontaneous regeneration.[2,3] This requires newly formed cementum and alveolar bone bridged by functional periodontal ligament. Conventional regenerative approaches aim at promoting the growth and differentiation of tissue-resident progenitor cells into fibroblasts, cementoblasts, and osteoblasts, while preventing the downgrowth of epithelial tissues into the periodontal defect. This approach, termed guided tissue

---

[a] Department of Clinical Dentistry, Faculty of Medicine - Tissue Engineering Group, University of Bergen, Årstadveien 19, 5009 Bergen, Norway; [b] Department of Immunology and Transfusion Medicine, Haukeland University Hospital, Jonas Lies vei 65, 5021 Bergen, Norway
* Corresponding author.
E-mail address: kamal.mustafa@uib.no

Dent Clin N Am 66 (2022) 111–130
https://doi.org/10.1016/j.cden.2021.06.004
0011-8532/22/© 2021 The Authors. Published by Elsevier Inc. This is an open access article under the CC BY-NC-ND license (http://creativecommons.org/licenses/by-nc-nd/4.0/).

dental.theclinics.com

regeneration, is represented by the application of barrier membranes with or without bioactive molecules such as enamel matrix derivative and recombinant growth factors.[4] Additionally, autogenous bone or bone substitutes of allogeneic, xenogeneic, or alloplastic origin, may be applied as scaffolds for cell growth and migration. These interventions have been shown to be effective clinically. However, a large heterogeneity among studies affirms the unpredictability of the treatments, and none of the existing treatment options have achieved complete periodontal regeneration.[5,6]

A conventional regenerative strategy, namely, bone grafting, mainly uses autogenous bone and various bone substitutes. Autogenous bone is considered as the golden standard because it has osteoconductive, osteoinductive, and osteogenic properties attributed to the components: autologous cells (eg, osteoblasts and their progenitor cells), extracellular matrix (ECM) components (eg, collagen, hydroxyapatite), and bioactive molecules (eg, bone morphogenetic protein-2 [BMP-2]).[7] However, owing to limitations in the amount of harvestable bone and the necessity of surgical intervention to donor sites, the use of allografts and xenografts, which are obtained from a donor of the same or different species, respectively, have been preferred as alternatives. Nevertheless, they carry the risk of unforeseen infection, disease transmission, and/or immune rejection.[8] In contrast, alloplastic or synthetic bone substitutes, which are mostly made from hydroxyapatite, for example, tricalcium phosphate, calcium sulfate, biphasic calcium phosphate, possess osteoconductivity, but are not of biological origin and, therefore, do not carry the risk of disease transmission. Bone substitute materials are delivered to osseous defects, including periodontal defects as scaffolds, and their osteoconductivity is hypothesized to stimulate endogenous progenitors to grow and differentiate into mature osteoblasts.[9] However, a systematic review has revealed that the outcome of periodontal therapy solely with bone grafting, that is, without accompanying barrier membranes, is predominantly ascribed to bone regeneration with an attachment of long junctional epithelium, but with a lack of newly formed cementum and periodontal ligament.[10] Moreover, the effect of such combinational therapies seems to be limited in horizontal and 2-walled intrabony defects, and inadequate in 3-walled intrabony and advanced furcation defects.[3]

Although conventional approaches to periodontal regeneration predominantly rely on the regenerative capacity of endogenous cells, the comparatively newer tissue engineering approach aims to combine exogeneous progenitor cells, biomaterial scaffolds, and bioactive molecules (signals) to address the complex architecture and function of the periodontal tissues.[11,12] In nature, ECM possesses optimal structural patterns and bioactivity, which regulate the growth and fate of the residing cells spatiotemporally. Meanwhile, the concept of biomimetics was brought into the fabrication of tissue engineered constructs for periodontal regeneration. Despite a large variance among studies, most of the designing concepts converge in mimicking the hierarchical organization of the native periodontal tissues, particularly the ECM, structurally and functionally in an ex vivo setting.[13] Scaffolds, therefore, serve as the core of tissue engineered construct because they offer 3-dimensional (3D) structural support and spatial guidance for cells. Moreover, their functionality may be further enhanced by incorporating bioactive molecules, for example, growth factors.[14] A wide variety of conventional and state-of-art scaffold fabrication methodologies such as decellularization, salt leaching, electrospinning, and 3D printing have been tested to fabricate biomimetic scaffolds to challenge the complex nature of periodontal tissues.[15] The aim of this article is to review the concepts of scaffold designing and fabrication, and to summarize the recent advancements in tissue engineering-based applications of biomimetic scaffolds for periodontal regeneration.

SCAFFOLD DESIGNING AND FABRICATION CONCEPT FOR PERIODONTAL REGENERATION

Scaffolds act as the core of tissue-engineered constructs because they offer spatio-temporal guidance for cells by providing architectural and biochemical clues.[14] Scaffold designing requires the selection of material, fabrication techniques, and functionalization methods (**Fig. 1**). This section summarizes scaffold designing and fabrication concept for periodontal applications.

Scaffold Architectures and Fabrication Techniques

Scaffolds provide the structural support and the guidance for exogenous and/or endogenous cells.[14] Generally, 3D scaffolds with high porosity and interconnectivity are preferable to achieve structural and functional restoration, because the architecture offers a suitable microenvironment for cell-to-cell interaction and scaffold-to-tissue integration at the implanted site.[15,16] In the early phase of implantation, the porous structures facilitate blood infiltration to the scaffolds and stabilize the blood clots, which is considered as a key initiator of tissue repair and regeneration through enriched vascularization.[17,18] Particularly, macropores ranging from 100 to 700 μm enhance vascularization at the implanted sites, whereas micropores of less than 100 μm may suppress cell growth owing to local ischemia.[16,19–22] High porosity also supports the diffusion of nutrients and gases as well as waste removal, which improves cellular metabolism and growth.[23–26] Various fabrication techniques have been used to design highly porous scaffolds.[15,27]

In nature, the ECM has an amorphous porous structure, acting as a scaffold. It regulates the recruitment, growth, and differentiation of resident cells via bioactive molecules, spatial patterning, and mechanical stimuli.[28] As an exogeneous complete form

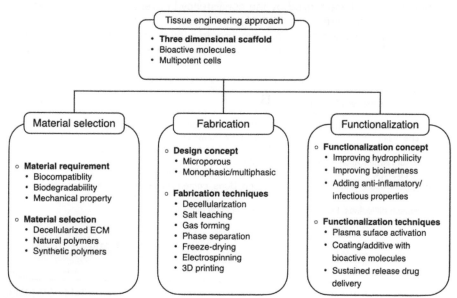

Fig. 1. Summary of scaffold designing and fabrication concept. Tissue engineering approach involves the combination of scaffolds, bioactive molecules, and multipotent cells. Scaffold functionality is determined by the selection of materials, fabrication methods, and functionalization techniques.

of ECM, decellularized ECM are widely applied to reproduce a 3D microenvironment at the implanted sites for tissue repair and regeneration. Decellularized ECM products from various origins, including human, porcine, or bovine dermis, and human amniotic membrane (hAM) are commercially available and used in clinical practice.[29] Recently, donor sites have been extended to the periodontal ligament itself, and attempts have been made to produce biomimetic periodontal scaffolds using decellularized ECM in combination with periodontal progenitor cells.[30–32] To reproduce the structural pattern of ECM artificially, various techniques have been translated into regenerative medicine. Salt leaching, gas forming, phase separation, and freeze drying are representative conventional methods to produce highly porous amorphous scaffolds (see the previous review on fabrication methods).[15] Salt leaching and gas forming techniques use salt and gas as porogen additives, whereas phase separation and freeze drying techniques use volatilization and sublimation of solvent and/or water in the polymer solution. Electrospinning is one of the representative engineering techniques used to produce fine fibrous scaffolds. It generates nonwoven nanoscaled-to-microscaled fibers, which reportedly mimic the native collagen fibrous network.[33–36] The electrospinning process requires a solvent–polymer mixture in a syringe pump, a collector, and a high voltage supply. When the high gradient of electric potential difference is applied between the metal syringe tip and the collector, electric charge accumulates on the polymer solution at the needle tip, and the polymer solution is ejected as a liquid jet toward the collector. When the jet reaches the collector, the polymer gets solidified because of evaporation of the solvent. These techniques allow for the fabrication of highly porous scaffolds, and resulting structures incorporate pores with various shapes and sizes, as if to recapitulate the structural pattern of the native ECM.[27] However, the controllability of internal architecture, that is, pore size, pore distribution, and pore orientation, is relatively low in comparison with rapid prototyping methods represented by 3D printing.[15] Furthermore, the resulting structures are considered as monophasic; it is characterized by the consistency in overall physical and chemical properties within the structures (**Fig. 2A**).

Provided that periodontal regeneration requires the hierarchical orientation of multiple tissues, a multiphasic design (ie, biphasic or triphasic) is considered to direct

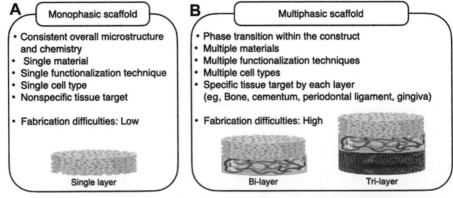

A Monophasic scaffold

- Consistent overall microstructure and chemistry
- Single material
- Single functionalization technique
- Single cell type
- Nonspecific tissue target

- Fabrication difficulties: Low

Single layer

B Multiphasic scaffold

- Phase transition within the construct
- Multiple materials
- Multiple functionalization techniques
- Multiple cell types
- Specific tissue target by each layer (eg, Bone, cementum, periodontal ligament, gingiva)

- Fabrication difficulties: High

Bi-layer   Tri-layer

Fig. 2. Summary of the characteristics of monophasic and multiphasic scaffolds. (*A*) Monophasic scaffolds consist of single layer with consistency in microstructural pattern and chemical property within the construct. (*B*) Multiphasic scaffolds are characterized by phasal transition within the construct. This includes the combination of different materials, functionalization techniques, and/or cell types.

progenitors to specific cell types more rigorously (**Fig.** 2B). This structure can be designed by layering components with different characteristics such as material composition, architectures, and functionalization.[27,37] Depending on designing concepts, countless combinations are possible. Although there is no perfect combination, a number of proof-of-concept studies have developed prototype designs that potentially favor the regeneration of the hierarchical structures.[37–44] In particular, 3D printing technology has recently emerged as a promising strategy to produce multilayered constructs for tissue engineering, because it overcomes the limitation of conventional fabrication techniques. Namely, difficulties in precise structural control and reproducibility are avoided. Moreover, recent advances in bioprinting have empowered the possibility of producing functional artificial organs in vitro.[45] With the help of 3D computer-aided design (CAD) modeling software, constructs can be built up in a layer-by-layer fashion in accordance with the blueprints. Currently, 3D printers for biomedical applications can achieve a minimum of 10 μm resolution with high accuracy.[46–48] The major advantage of 3D printing for scaffold fabrication is attributable to its designing flexibility. Controlling porosity, pore size, interconnectivity, and strand alignment pattern creates structural gradient within the construct, which may guide tissue orientation. The 3D printed scaffolds could be produced in a monophasic or multiphasic form depending on its design. Further advantage of 3D printing derives from its compatibility with diagnostic imaging equipment such as a cone beam computed tomography (CT) scan and intraoral 3D scanner. The geometry of periodontal defects is scanned and transferred into CAD modeling software to produce custom-designed 3D scaffolds adapting to the defect.[49] This personalized medicine approach is expected to increase the predictability of periodontal therapy for advanced tissue defects.

Polymeric Scaffold Materials and Functionalization

Material development and scaffold designing have been the major interest in biomaterial research for regenerative medicine.[11] Although natural ECM serves as the ideal scaffold in nature, particular attention has been paid to the generation of biomimetic scaffolds using polymeric biomaterials. Polymeric biomaterials possess biodegradability and biocompatibility, which allow the materials to be used for a wide range of medical application as implants for soft and hard tissue regeneration.[50] Polymeric biomaterials are categorized based on their origin: natural and synthetic polymers.

Natural polymers represented by proteins (eg, collagen, silk) and polysaccharides (eg, cellulose, alginate, chitosan) are often referred as the first biodegradable biomaterials applied in clinical settings.[51–53] They possess inherent bioactive properties that actively interact with cellular components. For example, integrin-binding ligands are presented on protein-based polymers, which regulate cell adhesion, migration, proliferation, and differentiation.[54] However, natural polymers generally lack mechanical stability, and their mechanical/biological properties may significantly vary depending on extraction procedures.[50] Furthermore, their high susceptibility to enzymatic degradation may result in disharmonized scaffold resorption and tissue remodeling.[55] Therefore, reinforcement with resilient materials such as fibers or hydroxyapatites is often considered.[56]

In contrast, synthetic polymers such as polylactic acid, polycaprolactone (PCL), and poly(DL-lactide-co-glycolide) present superior mechanical properties and formability for clinical use in a variety of applications in addition to decent biocompatibility and biodegradability. By altering molecular weight and chemical composition, favorable biodegradability and mechanical properties are delivered to the scaffold.[57] However, unlike natural polymers synthetic polymers are biologically inert, and their hydrophobic nature may hinder blood infiltration, which potentially prevents the scaffold from integrating to the implanted site.[58] To supplement the bioinertness of the synthetic polymers, functionalization using techniques such as plasma surface activation and the coating/additive of bioactive molecules are preferably performed.[33,59] These include ECM proteins (eg, collagen, fibronectin, gelatin),[59–61] growth factors (eg, BMP-2, BMP-7, fibroblast growth factor-2, and platelet-derived growth factor BB),[43,62–65] specialized proresolving mediators (eg, resolving D1),[66] and various types of antibiotics and anti-inflammatory drugs.[67–69] Generally, functionalization to the synthetic polymer does not alter the bulk property of the materials but increases interaction between material and tissues.[50] With this background in scaffold design and fabrication, the subsequent sections discuss the applications of various scaffold-based tissue engineering strategies in experimental settings for periodontal regeneration.

MONOPHASIC SCAFFOLD APPROACHES FOR PERIODONTAL REGENERATION
Decellularized Extracellular Matrix as an Exogeneous Natural Matrix

ECM is a natural form of complete scaffold, providing a suitable biochemical and biomechanical microenvironment for the residing cells. In a current clinical practice, an autologous connective tissue graft (CTG) is a frequent procedure to augment soft tissue. In addition to soft tissue regain, a histologic evaluation has revealed that CTG leads to the regeneration of cementum on the dentin surface, which may be bound to newly formed periodontal ligament, indicating connective tissue exhibits cementoconductivity.[70] However, the procedure is accompanied by a number of complications not only at the recipient site, but at the donor site such as pain, infection, bleeding, and necrosis.[71]

To overcome the limitation of the autologous soft tissue graft, decellularized ECM from allogenic or xenogeneic origin have been an alternative (**Fig. 3**). Acellular dermal matrix (ADM) from human skin is the most common decellularized ECM scaffold in periodontal treatment.[29] Although most of the clinical application in dentistry is limited to periodontal plastic surgery, its cementoconductivity and osteoconductivity supported by periodontal ligament regeneration has been suggested by in vivo models. A study using mini pigs with surgically created fenestration defects showed that clinical attachment gain by ADM was comparable with by CTG after 3 months of healing period, but ADM implantation led to greater new cementum regeneration with the narrower length of epithelial and connective tissue attachment.[72] The regenerative capacity of ADM may be further enhanced by combining bone substitute, as shown previously in beagle dogs that ADM in combination with beta-tricalcium phosphate induced the greater periodontal regeneration with thick cementum layers and alveolar bone formation that were bridged by periodontal ligament than ADM alone and coronally repositioned flap surgery.[73] Similarly, xenogeneic decellularized matrix possess comparable effects on the regeneration of periodontal tissue, although soft tissue response may differ.[72,74,75] There is a lack of evidence in the use of ADM to intrabony or furcation defects, but it supports the adhesion, robust proliferation of human periodontal ligament cells (PDLC) and possesses optimal biocompatibility and biodegradability for periodontal regeneration, suggesting its potency as a scaffold material.[76]

The hAM obtained from maternal donors undergoing caesarian section is another source of allogenic ECM, mainly for soft tissue repair and regeneration.[77] There is an absence of blood vessels and lymphatic tissue in hAM, and it has high durability and superior mechanical property attributed to the tight network of collagen and

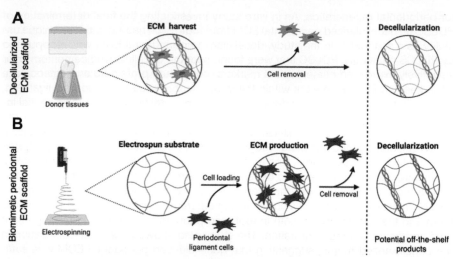

Fig. 3. Schematic illustration of the fabrication workflow of decellularized ECM scaffolds and biomimetic periodontal ECM scaffolds. (*A*) Decellularized ECM scaffolds are produced by harvesting ECM from donor sites such as dermis, amniotic membrane, and periodontal tissues followed by decellularization process. (*B*) Biomimetic periodontal ECM scaffolds are produced by the combination of nano-scaled electrospun substrate and allogenic PDLCs. The cells loaded on the substrate produce periodontal-specific ECM, which remains deposited after decellularization.

elastin fibers.[78] Human AM has been proven to contains rich growth factors such as epithelial growth factor, basic fibroblast growth factor, transforming growth factor-α and -β, vascular endothelial growth factor, and hepatocyte growth factor, all of which are positively corelated to periodontal regeneration through anti-inflammatory effects, immunomodulatory effects, antibacterial effects, and promotion of endogenous progenitor growth.[79–82] On hAM, PDLC are able to maintain their phenotype as in vivo with robust expression of ki-67, vimentin, desmoplakin, and ZO-1, but not keratins 4 and 13, suggesting its compatibility for periodontal regeneration.[70] It was shown that the use of hAM as a barrier membrane in combination with hydroxyapatite granules had advantageous effects on the suppression of the local inflammation at the recipient site, resulting in greater clinical attachment gain with increased bone generation than the bone substitutes only.[83,84] Although the efficacy of hAM alone to induce periodontal regeneration remains elusive, it was proven to be a promising scaffold for cell-based periodontal therapy.[85,86] An in vivo study in immunodeficient mice showed that hAM loaded with periodontal ligament stem cells (PDLSC) induced bone regeneration in surgically created class II furcation defects.[85] The histologic analysis confirmed new cementum formation, with single-layered cementblast-like cells on the surface, in which Sharpey's fibers were inserted. Similarly, the transplantation of adipose-derived mesenchymal stem cells on hAM regenerated 2-wall osseous defects in a rat model.[86] These results confirmed that hAM supported cementogenesis, osteogenesis, and fibrogenesis in experimental periodontal defects.

The ECM could also be obtained from dental tissues. Indeed, a detailed protocol to harvest and decellularize ECM from dental tissues without deteriorating intermingled collagen fiber networks have been recently reported, and it was successfully applied to periodontal tissues.[32,87] Naturally, the ECM of periodontal origin could be considered to possess the ideal microenvironment (eg, topography, protein composition) for periodontal regeneration. An in vitro study investigating the fatal determination of PDLSC on decellularized periodontal ECM from tooth slice has indicated its unique usability as a scaffold.[32] In the study, decellularized periodontal ECM was repopulated by PDLCS. Strikingly, PDLSC that were found near the decellularized cementum layer selectively expressed cementoblast markers, cementum protein-23 and osteocalcin, while keeping fibrous network within the decellularized area of periodontal ligament. This finding has confirmed that decellularized periodontal tissues maintains spatial information, which may guide the fate of PDLSC. Although no study has tested the regenerative capacity of decellularized periodontal EMC in periodontal defects, a tooth replantation model in beagle dogs has suggested that it potentially regenerates periodontal tissues structurally and functionally.[44] In the study, mandibular premolars were extracted and processed to decellularize the residual periodontal tissues on the root surface. The teeth were then replanted in the surgically expanded extraction socket. Interestingly, there was no significant difference between the freshly extracted teeth and the decellularized teeth in root resorption, recovered periodontal ligament area and new cementum formation. The study also showed rich revascularization in the decellularized matrix, suggesting that decellularized periodontal ECM was sufficient to retrieve its hierarchical structure and function by recruiting endogenous progenitors.

Nevertheless, the clinical translation of decellularized ECM originated from periodontal tissues seems challenging although periodontal ligament can be obtained from deciduous teeth, wisdom teeth, and extracted teeth for orthodontics treatment and then cryopreserved. The technique requires the provision of infrastructure, namely, "tooth banks," and improved cost efficiency before being manufactured as off-the-shelf products for example, ADM and hAM.[88]

Bioengineered Periodontal Extracellular Matrix as a Biomimetic Approach

Contrary to natural ECM-based approaches, bioengineering techniques may be used to produce biomimetic periodontal scaffolds in combination with progenitor cells and/ or bioactive molecules. A nanotopographical pattern of scaffolds, such as pores, grooves, and ridges, regulates cell growth, mobility, and fate.[89–91] Various techniques have been used to produce biomimetic ECM which has close resemblance to natural fibrous ECM. In particular, electrospinning has caught appreciable attention because of the unique features of the end products. Electrospun scaffolds consist of nonwoven nano-to-micro filaments with favorable porosity and interconnectivity for cell growth, which resemble to the structural pattern of natural ECM.[92] It is compatible with various natural and synthetic polymers, and further functionalization may be combined by adding bioactive molecules in the melts.[33]

Electrospun constructs have been used as a substrate to produce biomimetic periodontal ECM in combination with progenitor cells (**Fig. 2**B). Simply, PDLC seeded on an electrospun substrate were able to produce ECM by secreting collagen I, fibronectin, and rich growth factors, which are found in native periodontal tissues, such as basic fibroblast growth factor, vascular endothelial growth factor, and hepatocyte growth factor.[30,93] Importantly, the secreted proteins were preserved on the substrate after the decellularization process, indicating that the engineered construct mimicked the architecture and function of the native periodontal ECM.[30,31] Furthermore, the electrospun substrate provided a structural reinforcement during production process, which prevented the construct from being deformed and damaged during production process.[31] This allowed for further preclinical assessment of the biomimetic periodontal ECM in surgically created periodontal fenestration defects in rat, showing that it significantly promoted the regeneration of periodontal ligament, cementum, and alveolar bone in comparison to electrospun PCL scaffolds alone.[35] It has been shown that decellularized bioengineered ECM did not show immunogenicity, and it could be repopulated by allogenic and xenogeneic cells[30,35,93,94] Therefore, the concept of biomimetic periodontal ECM has a potential to be clinically transferred as off-the-shelf products.

The idea of biomimetic periodontal ECM may be further enhanced by controlling nanofiber orientation. On parallelly aligned PCL electrospun nanofibers, PDLC upregulated the expression of periostin, which regulates homeostasis of periodontal tissues in response to occlusal load.[95,96] Further in vivo observation in a periodontal fenestration defect model in rat showed that aligned PCL electrospun nanofibers loaded by PDLC noticeably regenerated periodontal ligament, which was perpendicularly oriented to the root surface, whereas randomly aligned nanofibers resulted in irregular ligament orientation.[96] This finding suggests that fiber orientation governs the architecture and function at the regenerated sites.

The functionalization of electrospun constructs may also expand the feasibility of hierarchical periodontal regeneration. For example, adding collagen type 1 and nanohydroxyapatites in PCL solution before extrusion allowed the end product to be osteoinductive, promoting the expression of alkaline phosphatase and osteocalcin expression by PDLCs.[97] Provided that periodontitis is an inflammatory disease caused by bacterial infection, functionalization with nonsteroidal anti-inflammatory drugs or antibiotics in anticipation of sustained drug release seems valid. The immobilization of nonsteroidal anti-inflammatory drugs such as meloxicam and ibuprofen in electrospun fibers allowed the construct to possess a long-term anti-inflammatory effect.[67–69] Interestingly, PCL electrospun scaffolds functionalized with ibuprofen selectively suppressed the proliferation of gingival cells subjected to *Porphyromonas gingivalis* lipopolysaccharide.[67] In an experimentally induced periodontitis model, PCL electrospun scaffolds functionalized with ibuprofen significantly decreased local inflammation and further progression but improved the clinical attachment level in comparison with the nonfunctionalized counterpart. Functionalization with antibiotics such as doxycycline hydrochloride, metronidazole, and tetracycline hydrochloride has been also suggested to be efficacious against the progression of periodontitis and to provide better sustainability after implantation.[98–100] These functionalization techniques do not alter the bulk properties of the polymeric scaffolds, but may offer additional benefits to periodontal regenerative therapy.[100]

MULTIPHASIC SCAFFOLD APPROACH FOR TARGETING TISSUE-SPECIFIC REGENERATION

Periodontal regeneration requires the spatiotemporal reorganization of newly formed periodontal ligament, cementum, and alveolar bone. These components are suggestive of porous medium with approximately 70% to 90% porosity, but each component has unique cellular components, matrix pattern, and functionality.[101–103] Therefore, multiphasic scaffolds are designed to consist of multiple components layer by layer, each of which specifically targets their corresponding tissue. There are countless designing concepts to achieve compartmentalized periodontal regeneration; it can be the combination of differential materials, architectural patterns, functionalization, and cell types.[37]

Biphasic scaffolds are often designed to combine bone compartment and periodontal compartment. Vaquette and colleagues (2012) developed double-layered PCL scaffolds which consisted of a bone compartment produced by 3D printing and an electrospun periodontal compartment.[38] In this study, osteoblasts in suspension and PDLC in sheet were loaded on their corresponding components, and then the construct was placed on a dentin block as the periodontal compartment was in contact with the dentin surface before subcutaneous transplantation in an immunodeficiency rat model. The histologic evaluation noted that a cementum-like tissue was formed on the dentin surface in which fibrous attachment supported, whereas the expression of alkaline phosphatase was promoted on the bone compartment side. The following study further optimized the scaffold design by functionalizing the bone compartment with calcium phosphates, showing improved bone formation.[39] The other common biphasic approach is to combine a barrier membrane and porous scaffold as one unit. Despite differences in designing concept among studies, it would be concluded the concept may improve the tissue regeneration in comparison with barrier membrane or scaffold alone.[40–42] However, further comparative studies between the biphasic scaffold approach and the conventional combination of barrier membrane and graft material separately are needed to verify its additional therapeutic benefit.

Triphasic scaffolds are mostly designed to individually target each of 3 components in periodontal tissues to provide more specific spaciotemporal guidance. Despite complexity in fabrication methods, several studies have successfully produced triphasic scaffolds for periodontal application. For example, 3D printing technology facilitates producing triphasic scaffolds by changing strand alignment patterns. Lee and colleagues[43] (2014) verified the triphasic concept by the orthodox tissue engineering approach, namely, by combining scaffolds, bioactive molecules, and progenitor cells. In this study, triphasic 3D printed scaffolds of nanohydroxyapatite-containing PCL were designed by changing porous patterns. Three phases were designed with 100 μm, 600 μm, and 300 μm microchannels to approach cementum/dentin interface, periodontal ligament, and alveolar bone, respectively. Subsequently, layers for the cementum–dentin interface, periodontal ligament, and alveolar bone were functionalized with human amelogenin, connective tissue growth factor, and BMP-2, respectively, before the scaffold was loaded by dental pulp stem cells and transplanted subcutaneously in immunodeficient mice. Notably, phase-specific tissue formation was observed: dense and polarized mineral formation with the upregulation of dentin sialophosphoprotein and cement matrix protein 1 in the cementum/dentin phase, aligned fibrous matrix formation with the upregulation of collagen type 1 in the periodontal ligament phase, and scattered mineral formation with the upregulation of bone sialoprotein in the bone phase. This finding suggests that multiphasic structures effectively guide tissue-specific regeneration by providing optimal microstructure and spatiotemporal delivery of bioactive molecules. Another example is the combination of differential cell types and mechanical properties. Varoni and colleagues[44] (2017) produced chitosan-based porous scaffolds that consisted of bone and periodontal layers produced by the freeze-drying method and a dense mesh gingival layers by electrochemical deposition. Differential stiffness was given to each of the layers by controlling molecular weight of cross-linking reagent: a stiff layer aiming for bone regeneration and a soft layer for the interaction with the gingiva and the periodontal ligament. Osteoblast, PDLC, and gingival fibroblast were then seeded to their corresponding layers. In an in vivo ectopic periodontal model, as expected, robust expression of tissue specific markers was found: periostin and collagen type 1 in the periodontal ligament layer, osteopontin and bone sialoprotein in the bone layer, and cement matrix protein-1 adjacent to the dentin surface. Also, putative cementum and bone were newly formed in the bone and periodontal layers.

It is also relevant to mention other studies that have introduced novel fabrication techniques for triphasic scaffolds that may potentially guide hierarchical regeneration, albeit without testing their in vivo efficacy.[37,104,105] Nevertheless, scaffold fabrication is complicated with each additional phase, particularly with regard to small scaffolds for periodontal applications, and a lack of in vivo evidence for the efficacy of such complex scaffolds precludes a conclusion on their current clinical relevance.

CUSTOM-DESIGNED 3-DIMENSIONAL SCAFFOLD FOR A PERSONALIZED PERIODONTAL APPROACH

A personalized medicine approach underlies the concept of pathologic variation among patients.[106] Optimal periodontal regeneration requires spatial guidance to progenitor cells with rich vascularization while preventing epithelial downgrowth.[107] Therefore, 3D scaffolds with defect-specific geometry may enhance periodontal regeneration. This goal could be achieved by applying a medical imaging system such as a high-resolution cone beam CT scan in scaffold designing. The prototype workflow of custom-designed 3D scaffolds for periodontal regeneration was introduced by Park and colleagues[49,63] (2010, 2012). Surgically created periodontal fenestration defects were scanned by a micro-CT scan, and the scanned files were then transferred into CAD software as 3D image data in .*stl* format, where the scaffold geometry was designed to adapt to the defect. In the scaffold, microchannel architectures were included in the scaffold to provide an orientational guide to periodontal ligament fibers. Subsequently, a wax mold was created by a wax printer, and PCL was casted in the mold.[49,63] After the sterilization process, PDLC were loaded on the custom-designed scaffold and transplanted to the defect site.[63] After 4 weeks of healing, the custom-designed scaffold resulted in a significant increase in bone mass and mineral density, and the alignment of regenerated periodontal ligament was oriented more regularly in comparison with amorphous scaffolds with random pores produced by the freeze-drying method. Strikingly, the expression of periostin, which is the regulator of collagen fibrogenesis found in functional periodontal ligament,[108] was evident in the treated site by the custom-designed scaffold, but not by the amorphous scaffold.[63] The development of high-resolution 3D printing technology has facilitated the fabrication of on-demand scaffolds (**Fig. 4**). The clinical implication of the approach was reported by Rasperini and colleagues[62] (2015) in which a fenestration defect in the mandibular canine was treated by 3D printed custom-designed scaffold. The scaffold was designed based on CT data and printed by selective laser sintering. During periodontal surgery, the scaffold was immersed in recombinant human platelet-derived growth factor BB and then transplanted in the defect site. After 12 months of the treatment, clinical attachment gain and radiological bone regeneration was observed without complication. In this case, however, the scaffold was exposed at 13 months, and then the entire scaffold was removed owing to infection. After histologic assessment and gel permeation chromatography showed that a great amount of the scaffold was still found with approximately 76% of PCL molecular weight remained. Also, the new bone formation was limited. This suggests that custom-designed scaffold may guide the tissue regeneration, but the prognosis largely depends on concordant material degradation and biological interaction between materials and tissues. Further optimization of internal microstructure, polymer selection, and polymer functionalization may contribute to an improved outcome.

Bioprinting technology has been emerging as a state-of-art tool to fabricate 3D biofunctional hierarchical architecture with one or multiple type(s) of living cell incorporated. It adds biological functionality to a conventional 3D printed scaffold because it mimics an in vivo cell-to-cell and cell-to matrix interaction within the construct. Currently, the technique has been used with trial-and-error steps to fabricate

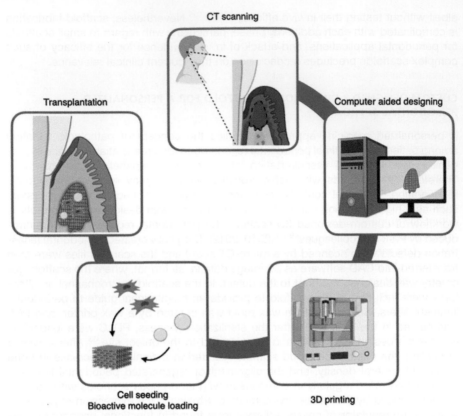

Fig. 4. Schematic illustration of the fabrication workflow of personalized 3D-printed scaffolds for periodontal regeneration. The geometry of periodontal defect obtained by CT scanning is processed in computer aided designing (CAD) software to design a scaffold which may adapt to the defect. Using CAD file, the scaffold is produced by 3D printing with a desired biomaterial. Multipotent cells and bioactive molecules may be incorporated to improve the functionality of the scaffold before transplantation.

bioartificial organs such as skin, bone, cartilage, liver, heart, kidney, lung, and nerve.[109] Owing to its immaturity, there are considerable challenges to overcome. These include the optimization of bioink, referring to a mixture of biomaterial and cells, and cytocompatible extrusion parameters.[109] For future application to periodontal regeneration, the optimization of bioink using PDLC has been just launched. By now, photocrosslinkable hydrogels, gelatin-methacryloyl and poly(ethylene glycol) dimethacrylate hydrogel were proposed as base materials, and the optimization of printability, mechanical stability, and cytocompatibility has been performed by testing different extrusion parameters and crosslinking methods.[110,111] The progress is in an early phase, but given the necessity of hierarchical regeneration, bioprinting in the field of periodontal regeneration is likely to gain more and more research attention.

CONCLUSION AND FUTURE IMPLICATIONS

Periodontal regeneration involves a high degree of complexity owing to the specialized nature and hierarchical structure of the periodontium. It requires a spatiotemporal coordination of both soft and hard tissues, namely gingival epithelium, periodontal ligament, cementum, and alveolar bone. Additionally, it is highly susceptible to oral microflora, and therefore controlling local inflection and inflammation determines the prognosis and therapeutic efficacy. Based on our current knowledge, the conventional grafting approach to periodontal defects with bone substitutes results in mainly bone regeneration with a long junctional epithelium regardless of material properties, and the regenerative potency of current therapies such as guided tissue regeneration and enamel matrix derivative is limited despite their clinical popularity. This warrants the necessity of further advancement in periodontal regenerative therapy based on the tissue engineering approach.

Indeed, tissue engineering in periodontics is a growing field: since the mid-1990s when its therapeutic potential was suggested, the number of studies has been exponentially increasing.[112] Advancement of material development, fabrication techniques, and digital solutions are remarkably propelling this novel approach to periodontal regeneration. Several studies have introduced prototypical scaffold designs that can potentially guide site-specific regeneration. This concept is based on the production of biomimetic periodontal scaffolds ex vivo by combining different materials and functionalization methods. The architectural patterns of scaffolds provide a spatial guidance to endogenous and exogeneous progenitor cells, whose functionality may be further enhanced by the inclusion of bioactive molecules on the scaffolds. Currently, high-resolution 3D printing technology allows for a rapid production of polymeric scaffolds in prescribed forms. The technique seems highly compatible with dental clinical settings where a CT scan and 3D intraoral scanner systems are now widely in use. This will allow to produce patient-specific scaffolds in a chair-side setting or in, for example, laboratories. Although clinical evidence for the efficacy of 3D-printed scaffolds is currently limited, further optimization of microstructure, material selection, and functionalization to add bioactive features may improve future clinical outcomes. Furthermore, advances in bioprinting technology may allow the production of patient-specific biomimetic periodontal implants.

Nevertheless, there is admittedly limited evidence on the advantage of the tissue engineering approach in comparison with the currently available treatment owing to the lack of in vivo and clinical evaluation in periodontal defect models. Challenges of preclinical testing notwithstanding, future studies should consider including more clinically relevant animal models of periodontitis, ideally in large animal models, to facilitate clinical translation. Furthermore, additional challenges, including compliance with good manufacturing practices and regulatory authorities must be overcome to facilitate the translation of novel tissue engineering therapies.[113] This involves the need for infrastructure improvements and quality control, with considerably higher costs of therapy as a consequence. Therefore, further investigations on clinical efficiency as well as cost effectiveness are required to validate the clinical applicability of tissue engineered constructs for periodontal regeneration.

CLINICS CARE POINTS

- Extracellular matrix obtained from periodontal ligament may be developed as off-the-shelf products.
- Biomimetic periodontal extracellular matrix can be produced by combining polymeric substrate and periodontal ligament-derived cells.
- Development of tooth-bank and stable provision of cell source are necessary for extracellular matrix approach.

- Multiphasic scaffolds may guide periodontal progenitor cells to specifically targeted cell types (i.e., fibroblasts, cementblasts, osteoblasts) despite difficulty in fabrication
- Defect-specific scaffolds produced by 3D printer may support periodontal regeneration for short-term, but there is currently no evidence on long-term prognosis
- Further in-vivo and clinical studies are needed to optimize scaffold design and material selection.

DISCLOSURE

The authors declare no potential conflict of interest.

ACKNOWLEDGMENTS

The authors gratefully acknowledge the Trond Mohn Foundation (Grant No. BFS2018TMT10) for financial support of this article.

REFERENCES

1. Gerritsen AE, Allen PF, Witter DJ, et al. Tooth loss and oral health-related quality of life: a systematic review and meta-analysis. Health Qual Life Outcomes 2010; 8:126.
2. Hughes FJ, Ghuman M, Talal A. Periodontal regeneration: a challenge for the tissue engineer? Proc Inst Mech Eng H 2010;224:1345–58.
3. Sculean A, Nikolidakis D, Schwarz F. Regeneration of periodontal tissues: combinations of barrier membranes and grafting materials - biological foundation and preclinical evidence: a systematic review. J Clin Periodontol 2008;35: 106–16.
4. Murphy KG, Gunsolley JC. Guided tissue regeneration for the treatment of periodontal intrabony and furcation defects. A systematic review. Ann Periodontol 2003;8:266–302.
5. Esposito M, Grusovin MG, Coulthard P, et al. Enamel matrix derivative (Emdogain) for periodontal tissue regeneration in intrabony defects. A Cochrane systematic review. Cochrane Database Syst Rev 2005;CD003875.
6. Needleman IG, V Worthington H, Giedrys-Leeper E, et al. Guided tissue regeneration for periodontal infra-bony defects. Cochrane Database Syst Rev 2006;CD001724.
7. Misch CM. Autogenous bone: is it still the gold standard? Implant Dent 2010; 19:361.
8. Eppley BL, Pietrzak WS, Blanton MW. Allograft and alloplastic bone substitutes: a review of science and technology for the craniomaxillofacial surgeon. J Craniofac Surg 2005;16:981–9.
9. Jimi E, Hirata S, Osawa K, et al. The current and future therapies of bone regeneration to repair bone defects. Int J Dent 2012;2012:1–7.
10. Sculean A, Nikolidakis D, Nikou G, et al. Biomaterials for promoting periodontal regeneration in human intrabony defects: a systematic review. Periodontol. 2000 2015;68:182–216.
11. Langer R, Vacanti JP. Tissue engineering. Science 1993;260:920–6.
12. Tollemar V, Collier ZJ, Mohammed MK, et al. Stem cells, growth factors and scaffolds in craniofacial regenerative medicine. Genes Dis 2016;3:56–71.
13. Green DW, Lee J-S, Jung H-S. Small-scale fabrication of biomimetic structures for periodontal regeneration. Front Physiol 2016;7:1–8.

14. O'Brien FJ. Biomaterials & scaffolds for tissue engineering. Mater Today 2011; 14:88–95.
15. Loh QL, Choong C. Three-dimensional scaffolds for tissue engineering applications: role of porosity and pore size. Tissue Eng B Rev 2013;19:485–502.
16. Karageorgiou V, Kaplan D. Porosity of 3D biomaterial scaffolds and osteogenesis. Biomaterials 2005;26:5474–91.
17. Tran PA. Blood clots and tissue regeneration of 3D printed dual scale porous polymeric scaffolds. Mater Lett 2021;285:129184.
18. Li Z, Lv X, Chen S, et al. Improved cell infiltration and vascularization of three-dimensional bacterial cellulose nanofibrous scaffolds by template biosynthesis. RSC Adv 2016;6:42229–39.
19. Hong WX, Hu MS, Esquivel M, et al. The role of hypoxia-inducible factor in wound healing. Adv Wound Care 2014;3:390–9.
20. Darby IA, Hewitson TD. Hypoxia in tissue repair and fibrosis. Cell Tissue Res 2016;553–62.
21. Klenke FM, Liu Y, Yuan H, et al. Impact of pore size on the vascularization and osseointegration of ceramic bone substitutes in vivo. J Biomed Mater Res A 2008;85A:777–86.
22. Murphy CM, O'Brien FJ. Understanding the effect of mean pore size on cell activity in collagen-glycosaminoglycan scaffolds. Cell Adhes Migr 2010;4:377–81.
23. Jin H, Zhuo Y, Sun Y, et al. Microstructure design and degradation performance in vitro of three-dimensional printed bioscaffold for bone tissue engineering. Adv Mech Eng 2019;11. 168781401988378.
24. Botchwey EA, Dupree MA, Pollack SR, et al. Tissue engineered bone: measurement of nutrient transport in three-dimensional matrices. J Biomed Mater Res 2003;67A:357–67.
25. Mastrullo V, Cathery W, Velliou E, et al. Angiogenesis in tissue engineering: As nature intended? Front Bioeng Biotechnol 2020;8:188.
26. Dutta RC, Dey M, Dutta AK, et al. Competent processing techniques for scaffolds in tissue engineering. Biotechnol Adv 2017;35:240–50.
27. Jeon JE, Vaquette C, Klein TJ, et al. Perspectives in multiphasic osteochondral tissue engineering. Anat Rec (Hoboken) 2014;297:26–35.
28. Nakayama KH, Hou L, Huang NF. Role of extracellular matrix signaling cues in modulating cell fate commitment for cardiovascular tissue engineering. Adv Healthc Mater 2014;3:628–41.
29. Tavelli L, McGuire MK, Zucchelli G, et al. Extracellular matrix-based scaffolding technologies for periodontal and peri-implant soft tissue regeneration. J Periodontol 2020;91:17–25.
30. Farag A, Vaquette C, Theodoropoulos C, et al. Decellularized periodontal ligament cell sheets with recellularization potential. J Dent Res 2014;93:1313–9.
31. Farag A, Vaquette C, Hutmacher DW, et al. Fabrication and characterization of decellularized periodontal ligament cell sheet constructs. Methods Mol Biol 2017;37:403–12.
32. Son H, Jeon M, Choi H-J, et al. Decellularized human periodontal ligament for periodontium regeneration. PLoS One 2019;14:e0221236.
33. Kurokawa N, Endo F, Maeda T, et al. Electrospinning and surface modification methods for functionalized cell scaffolds. In: Ficai D, Grumezescu AM, editors. Micro and Nano Technologies, Nanostructures for Novel Therapy. Elsevier; 2017. p. 201–25.
34. Lannutti J, Reneker D, Ma T, et al. Electrospinning for tissue engineering scaffolds. Mater Sci Eng C 2007;27:504–9.

35. Farag A, Hashimi SM, Vaquette C, et al. The effect of decellularized tissue engineered constructs on periodontal regeneration. J Clin Periodontol 2018;45: 586–96.
36. Cortez Tornello PR, Caracciolo PC, Igartúa Roselló JI, et al. Electrospun scaffolds with enlarged pore size: porosimetry analysis. Mater Lett 2018;227:191–3.
37. Ivanovski S, Vaquette C, Gronthos S, et al. Multiphasic scaffolds for periodontal tissue engineering. J Dent Res 2014;93:1212–21.
38. Vaquette C, Fan W, Xiao Y, et al. A biphasic scaffold design combined with cell sheet technology for simultaneous regeneration of alveolar bone/periodontal ligament complex. Biomaterials 2012;33:5560–73.
39. Costa PF, Vaquette C, Zhang Q, et al. Advanced tissue engineering scaffold design for regeneration of the complex hierarchical periodontal structure. J Clin Periodontol 2014;41:283–94.
40. Requicha JF, Viegas CA, Muñoz F, et al. A tissue engineering approach for periodontal regeneration based on a biodegradable double-layer scaffold and adipose-derived stem cells. Tissue Eng A 2014;20:2483–92.
41. Requicha JF, Viegas CA, Hede S, et al. Design and characterization of a biodegradable double-layer scaffold aimed at periodontal tissue-engineering applications. J Tissue Eng Regen Med 2016;10:392–403.
42. Carlo Reis EC, Borges APB, Araújo MVF, et al. Periodontal regeneration using a bilayered PLGA/calcium phosphate construct. Biomaterials 2011;32:9244–53.
43. Lee CH, Hajibandeh J, Suzuki T, et al. Three-dimensional printed multiphase scaffolds for regeneration of periodontium complex. Tissue Eng Part A 2014; 20:1342–51.
44. Varoni EM, Vijayakumar S, Canciani E, et al. Chitosan-based trilayer scaffold for multitissue periodontal regeneration. J Dent Res 2018;97:303–11.
45. Murphy SV, Atala A. 3D bioprinting of tissues and organs. Nat Biotechnol 2014; 32:773–85.
46. Liu F, Wang X. Synthetic polymers for organ 3D printing. Polymers (Basel) 2020; 12:1765.
47. Han T, Kundu S, Nag A, et al. 3D printed sensors for biomedical applications: a review. Sensors 2019;19:1706.
48. Derakhshanfar S, Mbeleck R, Xu K, et al. 3D bioprinting for biomedical devices and tissue engineering: a review of recent trends and advances. Bioact Mater 2018;3:144–56.
49. Park CH, Rios HF, Jin Q, et al. Biomimetic hybrid scaffolds for engineering human tooth-ligament interfaces. Biomaterials 2010;31:5945–52.
50. Tallawi M, Rosellini E, Barbani N, et al. Strategies for the chemical and biological functionalization of scaffolds for cardiac tissue engineering: a review. J R Soc Interf 2015;12:20150254.
51. Nair LS, Laurencin CT. Biodegradable polymers as biomaterials. Prog Polym Sci 2007;32:762–98.
52. Dhandayuthapani B, Yoshida Y, Maekawa T, et al. Polymeric scaffolds in tissue engineering application: a review. Int J Polym Sci 2011;2011:1–19.
53. Filippi M, Born G, Chaaban M, et al. Natural polymeric scaffolds in bone regeneration. Front Bioeng Biotechnol 2020;8:474.
54. Zhao J, Santino F, Giacomini D, et al. Integrin-targeting peptides for the design of functional cell-responsive biomaterials. Biomedicines 2020;8:307.
55. Banerjee A, Chatterjee K, Madras G. Enzymatic degradation of polymers: a brief review. Mater Sci Technol 2014;30:567–73.

56. Mano J, Silva G, Azevedo H, et al. Natural origin biodegradable systems in tissue engineering and regenerative medicine: present status and some moving trends. J R Soc Interf 2007;4:999–1030.
57. Heljak MK, Swieszkowski W, Kurzydlowski KJ. Modeling of the degradation kinetics of biodegradable scaffolds: the effects of the environmental conditions. J Appl Polym Sci 2014;131:40280.
58. Baican M, Stoleru E, Vasile C. Cellular response to synthetic polymers. In: Mozafari M, editor. Woodhead Publishing Series in Biomaterials, Handbook of Biomaterials Biocompatibility. Woodhead Publishing; 2020. p. 269–319.
59. Campos DM, Gritsch K, Salles V, et al. Surface entrapment of fibronectin on electrospun PLGA scaffolds for periodontal tissue engineering. Biores Open Access 2014;3:117–26.
60. Liu Z, Yin X, Ye Q, et al. Periodontal regeneration with stem cells-seeded collagen-hydroxyapatite scaffold. J Biomater Appl 2016;31:121–31.
61. Carmagnola D, Tarce M, Dellavia C, et al. Engineered scaffolds and cell-based therapy for periodontal regeneration. J Appl Biomater Funct Mater 2017;15: e303–12.
62. Rasperini G, Pilipchuk SP, Flanagan CL, et al. 3D-printed bioresorbable scaffold for periodontal repair. J Dent Res 2015;94:153S–7S.
63. Park CH, Rios HF, Jin Q, et al. Tissue engineering bone-ligament complexes using fiber-guiding scaffolds. Biomaterials 2012;33:137–45.
64. Vasconcelos DP, Costa M, Neves N, et al. Chitosan porous 3D scaffolds embedded with resolvin D1 to improve in vivo bone healing. J Biomed Mater Res Part A 2018;106:1626–33.
65. Nakamura S, Ito T, Okamoto K, et al. Acceleration of bone regeneration of horizontal bone defect in rats using collagen-binding basic fibroblast growth factor combined with collagen scaffolds. J Periodontol 2019;90:1043–52.
66. Van Dyke TE. Pro-resolving mediators in the regulation of periodontal disease. Mol Aspects Med 2017;58:21–36.
67. Batool F, Morand D-N, Thomas L, et al. Synthesis of a novel electrospun polycaprolactone scaffold functionalized with ibuprofen for periodontal regeneration: an in vitro and in vivo study. Materials (Basel) 2018;11:580.
68. Yar M, Farooq A, Shahzadi L, et al. Novel meloxicam releasing electrospun polymer/ceramic reinforced biodegradable membranes for periodontal regeneration applications. Mater Sci Eng C 2016;64:148–56.
69. Farooq A, Yar M, Khan AS, et al. Synthesis of piroxicam loaded novel electrospun biodegradable nanocomposite scaffolds for periodontal regeneration. Mater Sci Eng C 2015;56:104–13.
70. Goldstein M, Boyan BD, Cochran DL, et al. Human histology of new attachment after root coverage using subepithelial connective tissue graft. J Clin Periodontol 2001;28:657–62.
71. Aguirre-Zorzano L-A, García-De La Fuente AM, Estefanía-Fresco R, et al. Complications of harvesting a connective tissue graft from the palate. A retrospective study and description of a new technique. J Clin Exp Dent 2017;9:e1439–45.
72. Núñez J, Caffesse R, Vignoletti F, et al. Clinical and histological evaluation of an acellular dermal matrix allograft in combination with the coronally advanced flap in the treatment of miller class I recession defects: an experimental study in the mini-pig. J Clin Periodontol 2009;36:523–31.
73. Okubo N, Fujita T, Ishii Y, et al. Coverage of gingival recession defects using acellular dermal matrix allograft with or without beta-tricalcium phosphate. J Biomater Appl 2013;27:627–37.

74. de Carvalho Formiga M, Nagasawa MA, Moraschini V, et al. Clinical efficacy of xenogeneic and allogeneic 3D matrix in the management of gingival recession: a systematic review and meta-analysis. Clin Oral Investig 2020;24:2229–45.

75. Aragoneses J, Suárez A, Rodríguez C, et al. Histomorphometric comparison between two types of acellular dermal matrix grafts: a mini pig animal model study. Int J Environ Res Public Health 2021;18:3881.

76. Guo J, Chen H, Wang Y, et al. A novel porcine acellular dermal matrix scaffold used in periodontal regeneration. Int J Oral Sci 2013;5:37–43.

77. Leal-Marin S, Kern T, Hofmann N, et al. Human amniotic membrane: a review on tissue engineering, application, and storage. J Biomed Mater Res B Appl Biomater 2020;109(8):1198–215.

78. Mamede AC, Botelhoeditors MF. Amniotic membrane. Dordrecht: Springer Netherlands; 2015.

79. Koizumi N, Inatomi T, Sotozono C, et al. Growth factor mRNA and protein in preserved human amniotic membrane. Curr Eye Res 2000;20:173–7.

80. Bosshardt DD, Schroeder HE. Cementogenesis reviewed: a comparison between human premolars and rodent molars. Anat Rec 1996;245:267–92.

81. Howell TH, Martuscelli G, Oringer J. Polypeptide growth factors for periodontal regeneration. Curr Opin Periodontol 1996;3:149–56.

82. Ferenczy PAH, de Souza LB. Comparison of the preparation and preservation techniques of amniotic membrane used in the treatment of ocular surface diseases. Rev Bras Oftalmol 2020;79:71–80.

83. Adachi K, Amemiya T, Nakamura T, et al. Human periodontal ligament cell sheets cultured on amniotic membrane substrate. Oral Dis 2014;20:582–90.

84. Kumar A, Chandra RV, Reddy AA, et al. Evaluation of clinical, antiinflammatory and antiinfective properties of amniotic membrane used for guided tissue regeneration: a randomized controlled trial. Dent Res J (Isfahan) 2015;12:127–35.

85. Iwasaki K, Komaki M, Yokoyama N, et al. Periodontal regeneration using periodontal ligament stem cell-transferred amnion. Tissue Eng Part A 2013;20.131209065021003.

86. Wu P-H, Chung H-Y, Wang J-H, et al. Amniotic membrane and adipose-derived stem cell co-culture system enhances bone regeneration in a rat periodontal defect model. J Formos Med Assoc 2016;115:186–94.

87. Song JS, Takimoto K, Jeon M, et al. Decellularized human dental pulp as a scaffold for regenerative endodontics. J Dent Res 2017;96:640–6.

88. Zeitlin BD. Banking on teeth – stem cells and the dental office. Biomed J 2020;43:124–33.

89. Wang WY, Pearson AT, Kutys ML, et al. Extracellular matrix alignment dictates the organization of focal adhesions and directs uniaxial cell migration. APL Bioeng 2018;2:046107.

90. Janson IA, Putnam AJ. Extracellular matrix elasticity and topography: material-based cues that affect cell function via conserved mechanisms. J Biomed Mater Res Part A 2015;103:1246–58.

91. Ermis M, Antmen E, Hasirci V. Micro and nanofabrication methods to control cell-substrate interactions and cell behavior: a review from the tissue engineering perspective. Bioact Mater 2018;3:355–69.

92. Wang X, Ding B, Li B. Biomimetic electrospun nanofibrous structures for tissue engineering. Mater Today 2013;16:229–41.

93. Jiang Y, Liu J-M, Huang J-P, et al. Regeneration potential of decellularized peri-odontal ligament cell sheets combined with 15-deoxy-Δ 12,14 -prostaglandin J 2 nanoparticles in a rat periodontal defect. Biomed Mater 2021;16:045008.

94. Heng BC, Zhu S, Xu J, et al. Effects of decellularized matrices derived from peri-odontal ligament stem cells and SHED on the adhesion, proliferation and oste-ogenic differentiation of human dental pulp stem cells in vitro. Tissue Cell 2016; 48:133–43.

95. Rios HF, Ma D, Xie Y, et al. Periostin is essential for the integrity and function of the periodontal ligament during occlusal loading in mice. J Periodontol 2008;79: 1480–90.

96. Yang M, Gao X, Shen Z, et al. Gelatin-assisted conglutination of aligned poly-caprolactone nanofilms into a multilayered fibre-guiding scaffold for periodontal ligament regeneration. RSC Adv 2019;9:507–18.

97. Wu X, Miao L, Yao Y, et al. Electrospun fibrous scaffolds combined with nano-scale hydroxyapatite induce osteogenic differentiation of human periodontal lig-ament cells. Int J Nanomedicine 2014;9:4135.

98. Jia L, Zhang X, Xu H, et al. Development of a doxycycline hydrochloride-loaded electrospun nanofibrous membrane for GTR/GBR applications. J Nanomater 2016;2016:1–10.

99. Verma P, Chaturvedi T, Gupta V, et al. Evaluation of metronidazole nanofibers in patients with chronic periodontitis: a clinical study. Int J Pharm Investig 2012; 2:213.

100. Ranjbar-Mohammadi M, Zamani M, Prabhakaran MP, et al. Electrospinning of PLGA/gum tragacanth nanofibers containing tetracycline hydrochloride for peri-odontal regeneration. Mater Sci Eng C 2016;58:521–31.

101. Bergomi M, Cugnoni J, Galli M, et al. Hydro-mechanical coupling in the peri-odontal ligament: a porohyperelastic finite element model. J Biomech 2011; 44:34–8.

102. Ortún-Terrazas J, Cegoñino J, Santana-Penín U, et al. Approach towards the porous fibrous structure of the periodontal ligament using micro-computerized tomography and finite element analysis. J Mech Behav Biomed Mater 2018;79:135–49.

103. Ho SP, Yu B, Yun W, et al. Structure, chemical composition and mechanical properties of human and rat cementum and its interface with root dentin. Acta Biomater 2009;5:707–18.

104. Shah AT, Zahid S, Ikram F, et al. Tri-layered functionally graded membrane for po-tential application in periodontal regeneration. Mater Sci Eng C 2019;103:109812.

105. Sprio S, Campodoni E, Sandri M, et al. A graded multifunctional hybrid scaffold with superparamagnetic ability for periodontal regeneration. Int J Mol Sci 2018; 19:3604.

106. Hamburg MA, Collins FS. The path to personalized medicine. N Engl J Med 2010;301–4.

107. Ramseier CA, Rasperini G, Batia S, et al. Advanced reconstructive technologies for periodontal tissue repair. Periodontol. 2000 2012;59:185–202.

108. Wen W, Chau E, Jackson-Boeters L, et al. TGF-β1 and FAK regulate periostin expression in PDL fibroblasts. J Dent Res 2010;89:1439–43.

109. Matai I, Kaur G, Seyedsalehi A, et al. Progress in 3D bioprinting technology for tissue/organ regenerative engineering. Biomaterials 2020;226:119536.

110. Thattaruparambil Raveendran N, Vaquette C, Meinert C, et al. Optimization of 3D bioprinting of periodontal ligament cells. Dent Mater 2019;35:1683–94.

111. Ma Y, Ji Y, Huang G, et al. Bioprinting 3D cell-laden hydrogel microarray for screening human periodontal ligament stem cell response to extracellular matrix. Biofabrication 2015;7:044105.
112. Bell E. Strategy for the selection of scaffolds for tissue engineering. Tissue Eng 1995;1:163–79.
113. Giancola R, Bonfini T, Iacone A. Cell therapy: cGMP facilities and manufacturing. Muscles Ligaments Tendons J 2012;2:243–7.

Nanomedicine and Periodontal Regenerative Treatment

Olivier Huck, DDS, PhD[a,b,c],*, Céline Stutz, PharmD, MSc[a],
Pierre-Yves Gegout, DDS, MSc[a,b,c], Hayriye Özçelik, PhD[a],
Nadia Benkirane-Jessel, PhD[a], Catherine Petit, DDS, MSc[a,b,c],
Fareeha Batool, PhD[a,b]

KEYWORDS

• Periodontitis • Nanomedicine • Nanocarriers • Inflammation • Biomaterials

KEY POINTS

• Nanomedicine is a promising tool to improve periodontal treatment outcomes with a decreased risk of side effects.
• Nanocarriers are able to deliver antibacterial, anti-inflammatory and proregenerative drugs or molecules.
• Nanoparticles or nanoreservoirs can be included in scaffolds, such as gels, membranes, and bone scaffolds.

INTRODUCTION

The regeneration of periodontal tissues is the ultimate goal of periodontal therapy. Despite impressive progress over the last 30 years, especially in terms of nonsurgical and surgical therapies (antibiotics, photodynamic therapy, probiotics, minimally invasive surgical approaches, biomaterials development, etc),[1–5] tissue regeneration remains difficult to achieve in some specific clinical scenario, such as complex lesions with a lack of bone walls or those that are difficult to reach, such as a furcation area. Pharmacologic approaches have been proposed to optimize treatment outcomes, targeting either infection, inflammation, or tissue growth. However, systemic administration is complex because it induces an unnecessary systemic loading of

[a] INSERM (French National Institute of Health and Medical Research), UMR 1260, Regenerative Nanomedicine, Fédération de Médecine Translationnelle de Strasbourg (FMTS), CRBS, 1 rue Eugène Boeckel, 67000 Strasbourg, France; [b] Université de Strasbourg, Faculté de Chirurgie-dentaire, 8 rue Sainte-Elisabeth, 67000 Strasbourg, France; [c] Pôle de médecine et chirurgie bucco-dentaire, Hôpitaux Universitaires de Strasbourg, Periodontology, 1 place de l'Hopital, 67000, Strasbourg, France
* Corresponding author. 8 rue Sainte-Elisabeth, 67000 Strasbourg, France.
E-mail address: o.huck@unistra.fr

Dent Clin N Am 66 (2022) 131–155
https://doi.org/10.1016/j.cden.2021.06.005
0011-8532/22/© 2021 Elsevier Inc. All rights reserved.

the drug as well as a decreased bioavailability at the periodontal pocket site.[6,7] To overcome such limitations and improve treatment outcomes, innovative nanotechnologies have been developed and tested over the last years with promising results. Nanomedicine has been defined as "the monitoring, repair, construction, and control of human biological systems at the molecular level, using engineered nanodevices and nano-structures."[8] It uses the properties of materials at a nanometric scale to improve diagnosis and imaging, as well as to promote tissue regeneration through the delivery of bioactive compounds or drugs.

The application of nanomedicine and nanotechnologies has been suggested to be a part of the therapeutic arsenal for several diseases such as cancers[9] and inflammatory diseases such as rheumatoid arthritis,[10] aiming to deliver most efficiently the drug or active compounds to a specific site. Therefore, the use of such nanotechnologies for the treatment of periodontal diseases, mainly periodontitis, has been proposed with the goal to deliver a sufficient concentration of active molecules at the targeted site and to avoid its distribution in nonspecific tissues, consequently decreasing the risk of side effects. The onset and development of the periodontal lesion involve several cell types, including epithelial cells from the junctional epithelium, fibroblasts from the connective tissue, bone cells, and all immune cells, especially polymorphonuclear neutrophils and macrophages.[11–13] The targeting of such cells to arrest the proinflammatory host response and/or to promote the proresolution of the inflammation is then required and several nanocarriers have been developed. Nanocarriers are polymers of biological or synthetic origin that are used to deliver drugs such as antibiotics, antibodies, or other macromolecules adsorbed on their surfaces or within their core and are for most of them biodegradable. Indeed, chitosan, polylactic-co-glycolic acid (PLGA), carbon quantum dots, and mesoporous silica/bioactive glass have been developed and tested in several applications including periodontitis[14,15] (**Fig. 1**). The aim of this review is to describe the advantages of such nanoparticles and the feasibility of their use in the specific context of periodontitis treatment.

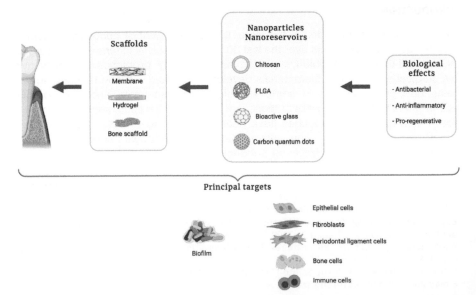

Fig. 1. Nanomedicine strategies designed for periodontal treatment. Nanoparticles/nanoreservoirs could be implemented in different scaffolds to display their antibacterial, anti-inflammatory, and proregenerative properties with a low risk of systemic side effects.

CHITOSAN-BASED NANOMATERIALS

Chitosan is a natural polysaccharide that can be easily produced via the alkaline N-deacetylation process of a natural biopolymer commonly found in the shells of marine crustaceans and in fungi cells walls, the chitin.[16] It is widely used to synthesize biomedical scaffolds or implants owing to its biocompatibility, antibacterial properties, positive host response, and sufficient mechanical strength.[17] It is already used as a wound dressing due to its interesting hemostatic and antimicrobial properties contributing to the formation of the blood clot and to a decrease in the risk of infection at the treated site.[18,19] The inherent antimicrobial properties of chitosan, mainly associated with its cationic nature, have been demonstrated against different microorganisms in several cellular and animal models. In the context of periodontitis, the antibacterial properties of chitosan nanoparticles have been tested against major periodontal pathogens such as *Porphyromonas gingivalis* and *Aggregatibacter actinomycetemcomitans*. Indeed, it was shown that exposure of these bacteria to chitosan nanoparticles inhibits bacterial growth in vitro.[20] Chitosan-based nanoparticles could also be loaded with antimicrobial peptide to interact with pathogens in a planktonic state, as well as when organized in biofilms as observed for *P.gingivalis*, *Fusobacterium nucleatum*, and *Streptococcus gordonii*.[21] It can also be loaded with drugs such as antibiotics, that is, minocycline and antiseptics such as chlorhexidine to enhance their properties.[22,23] Chitosan nanoparticles or nanoreservoirs have also been used to deliver on site immune-modulatory molecules and proregenerative factors. Several studies have been conducted in this regard with significant effects[24,25] (**Table 1**). For instance, the delivery of statins using chitosan carriers was evaluated and showed promising results in terms of periodontal regeneration. In a model of experimental periodontitis in dogs[26] or in a mouse calvarial defect.[27] Chitosan has also been used to synthesize nanoreservoirs that could be constructed on the fibers of scaffolds such as membrane. Such technology demonstrated efficiency toward the delivery of growth factors such as BMP-2 enhancing bone regeneration with improved biocalcification of the scaffold[25] and especially in the context of maxillary bone regeneration[28] (**Fig. 2**).

POLYLACTIC-CO-GLYCOLIC ACID

PLGA is a synthetic biodegradable copolymer widely used in medical applications owing to its minimal cytotoxicity.[39] Its degradation by hydrolysis results in biocompatible byproducts, lactic acid and glycolic acid, that are physiologically metabolized. PLGA has been used as a nanocarrier to deliver active drugs to treat several diseases or to promote tissue regeneration. It has been used extensively to design scaffolds, including barrier membranes, bone scaffolds, sponges, and gels[40] (**Fig. 3**). PLGA displays interesting physical properties because its viscosity is modulable; however, it is also associated with an initial burst release of the active molecule, and therefore is often use in combination with chitosan in a core shell technique.[41] The modulation of the thickness of the shell could be interesting to increase the time needed to deliver the active molecule. In the context of periodontal treatment, PLGA nanoparticles (or PLGA–chitosan nanoparticles) have already been tested in several model (in vitro and in vivo) and in clinical settings (**Table 2**). Indeed, antibiotics, compounds of natural origin with anti-inflammatory properties such as curcumin, metals such as silver, and immunomodulatory drugs such as statins have been loaded. Most of the studies exhibited positive outcomes resulting in a decrease in a decrease of periodontal pathogens growth and inflammatory cytokine secretion. Interestingly, PLGA nanoparticles have also been tested as methylene

Table 1
Representative studies evaluating potential use of CS nanoparticles in the context of periodontal treatment

Study	Type of Study	Active Drug	Size of Particles	Effects
Hu et al, 2021[21]	In vitro: biofilm (F nucleatum, P gingivalis and S gordonii)	Nal-P-113 (antimicrobial peptide) loaded poly (ethylene glycol) combined CS nanoparticles (Nal-P-113-PEG-CSNPs)	216.2 ± 1.6 nm	Prepared NPs inhibited the growth of F nucleatum, S gordonii, and P gingivalis
Soe et al, 2020[29]	In vitro: HPDLCs	AS loaded SBEβCD/CS NPs	25–350 nm	No cytotoxic effects to HPDCLs
Xu et al, 2020[30]	In vitro: effect of P gingivalis on HGFs	Dox:CS/CMCS-NPs	203.1 ± 10.51 nm	P gingivalis is strongly inhibited by Dox:CS/CMCS-NPs. Dox:CS/CMCS-NPs downregulated both gene and protein levels of NLRP3 inflammasome and IL-1β in HGFs
Martin et al, 2019[23]	In vitro: P gingivalis LPS-stimulated culture of HGF	MH-NPs	50 ± 17 nm	Expression levels of inflammation-related markers (IL-1b, TNFα, CXCL-8, NFKB1) significantly reduced after MH-NPs exposure
Aminu et al, 2019[31]	In vivo: experimental periodontitis in rat	Triclosan and flurbiprofen loaded in a CS-based hydrogel	100–400 nm	Antibacterial and anti-inflammatory effects of the CS-based hydrogel
Xue et al, 2019[32]	In vitro: Effect on proliferation and mineralization of periodontal membrane cells In vivo: Proliferation and mineralization of periodontal membrane cells were investigated	CS, PLGA, and silver nanoparticles (PLGA nanoparticles, CS nanoparticles, silver nanoparticles)	112–180 nm	No cytotoxicity and promotion of cell mineralization by the nanoparticles CS nanoparticles and silver nanoparticles in low concentrations showed antibacterial activity PLGA nanoparticles and CS nanoparticles complex in 3:7 ratio contributed to cell

	Test	Material	Size	Results
	and tested in animals (New Zealand White rabbits)			mineralization and had no cytotoxicity PLGA nanoparticles/CS nanoparticles/silver nanoparticles complex, which had the optimal proportion of the 3 materials, showed no cytotoxicity and contributed to cell mineralization
Hu et al, 2018[33]	In vitro: Cytocompatibility and biocompatibility in human periodontal ligament fibroblasts. Inhibition test on mixed bacteria (P gingivalis and Prevotella intermedia) In vivo: Test on biofilm formation and alveolar bone absorption (rats)	Quaternary ammonium CS, that is, TMC-Lip-DOX NPs	129.7 nm	TMC-Lip-DOX NPs achieved a great inhibition of free mixed bacteria and biofilm formation TMC-Lip-DOX NPs showed a good biocompatibility with human periodontal ligament fibroblasts NPs strongly inhibited biofilm formation and prevented alveolar bone absorption in vivo
He et al, 2018[34]	In vitro: cell culture of rBMSCs	Gln and CS composite GBR membrane containing hydroxyapatite nanoparticles and antimicrobial peptide-loaded PLGA microspheres		Gln/CS composite membrane had an ideal biocompatibility with good cell adhesion, spreading, and proliferation Gln/CS membrane-containing hydroxyapatite nanoparticles could promote osteogenic differentiation of rBMSCs Composite GBR membrane containing antimicrobial peptide-loaded PLGA microspheres exhibited a long-term sustained release of

(continued on next page)

Table 1
(continued)

Study	Type of Study	Active Drug	Size of Particles	Effects
				antimicrobial peptide, which had bactericidal activity within 1 week and antibacterial activity for up to 1 month against 2 kinds of bacteria, *S aureus* and *E coli*
Guarino et al, 2017[35]	In vitro: Inhibitory activity evaluated against *E coli*, *S aureus*, and *A actinomycetemcomitans*	Amoxicilline trihydrate loaded in CS nano-reservoirs	0.1–0.4 μm	Antibiotics such as amoxicilline trihydrate can be administered via PCL nanofibers decorated by drug loaded CS nanoparticles to decrease bacterial activity
Lin et al, 2017[36]	In vivo: Effect of nanosphere in induced periodontitis in rat	PLGA and CS encapsulated metronidazole and N-phenacylthiazolium bromide	499 ± 21.24 nm	Progression of periodontal bone loss significantly reduced in group N-phenacylthiazolium bromide at day 21 In groups metronidazole and N-phenacylthiazolium bromide, inflammation was significantly decreased
Li et al, 2017[37]	In vivo: In rat calvarial defect and periodontitis induced bony defect in beagle dog	pDNA-BMP2-loaded in CS nanoparticles (pDNA-BMP2)-GP		CS nanoparticles (pDNA-BMP2)-GP enhanced new bone formation in rat calvarial defects and enhanced bony defect healing in beagle dogs
Li et al, 2016[38]	In vitro: Release and cytocompatibility to HPDLCs	CSn loaded with pDNA-BMP2 into a CS-based hydrogel with α,β-glycerophosphate	270.1 nm	pDNA-BMP2 demonstrated a good cytocompatibility with HPDLCs and improved the cell growth

Author/Year	Description	Nanoparticle	Size	Findings
Lee et al, 2016[26]	In vitro: Cytotoxic effect and alkaline phosphatase activity of the nanoparticles in osteoblast cell culture and antibacterial activity against periodontal pathogens (A actinomycetemcomitans and Prevotella nigrescens) In vivo: Regeneration potential in 3 wall defect in beagle dog	PLGA-lovastatin-CS-tetracycline nanoparticles	111.5 nm.	PLGA-lovastatin-CS-tetracycline nanoparticles showed good biocompatibility, antibacterial activity, and increased alkaline phosphatase activity. A significantly increased new bone formation was found in defects filled with nanoparticles in dogs
Barreras et al, 2016[22]	In vitro: Antibacterial effect against Enterococcus faecalis cultures and infected collagen membranes	CS nanoparticles containing chlorhexidine	70.67 ± 14.86 nm	CS nanoparticles acted synergistically with chlorhexidine, inhibiting and eliminating significantly a greater amount of colony former units in both BHI-agar cultures and infected collagen membranes
Arancibia et al, 2013[20]	In vitro: Antibacterial effect against periodontal pathogens (P gingivalis, A actinomycetemcomitans) and inflammatory response in gingival fibroblasts	CS	Not specified	The growth of periodontal pathogens was inhibited at 5 mg/mL. CS exerts a predominantly anti-inflammatory activity by modulating PGE2 levels through the JNK pathway

Abbreviations: AS, asiaticoside; CMCS, carboxymethyl chitosan; CS, chitosan; Dox:CS/CMCS-NPs, doxycycline carried by NPs comprising CS/CMCS; Gln, Gelatin; HGF, human gingival fibroblasts; HPDLC, human periodontal ligament cell; LPS, lipopolysaccharide; MH-NPs; chitosan-nanoparticles loaded with minocycline; pDNA-BMP2; bone morphogenetic protein-2 plasmid DNA; PLGA, polylactide-glycolic acid co-polymer; rBMSCs, rat bone marrow mesenchymal stem cells; SBEβCD/CS NPs, sulfobutylether β-CD/chitosan nanoparticles; TMC-Lip-DOX NPs, N,N-trimethyl chitosan, a liposome, and doxycycline; TNF, tumor necrosis factor.

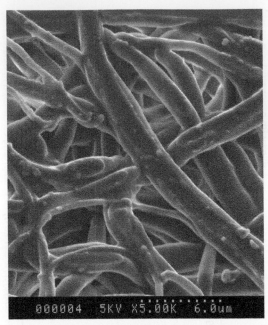

Fig. 2. Chitosan nanoreservoirs containing BMP-2 in polycaprolactone fibers.

blue carrier in the context of treatment of periodontal pockets with photodynamic therapy.[42,43] The use of nanocarriers, such as PLGA, allows to deliver locally a high concentration of photosensitizer at the site, decreasing the risk of multidrug resistance.[42]

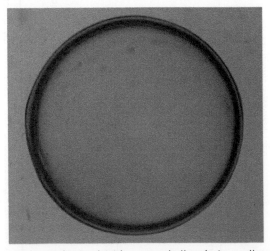

Fig. 3. PLGA nanoparticle synthesized with a core-shell technique allowing the loading of an active drug in the core of the particle.

Table 2
Representative studies evaluating potential use of PLGA nanoparticles in the context of periodontal treatment

Study	Type of Study	Active Drug	Size of Particles	Effects
Beg et al, 2020[44]	In vivo: experimental periodontitis in rats. Effect of in situ gel containing nanoparticle of moxifloxacin hydrochloride	Moxifloxacin hydrochloride	204.63–292.81 nm	Histopathologic studies demonstrated almost complete recovery after 3 wk of treatment. Results were better in moxifloxacin nanoparticles treated group vs commercially available gel (0.5% chlorhexidine and 1.5% metronidazole)
Ghavimi et al, 2020[45]	In vitro: *Staphylococcus aureus*, *Escherichia coli*, and *Enterococcus faecalis* cultures; Dental pulp stem cells. In vivo: alveolar bone defect in mongrel dogs. Antibacterial, cytocompatibility and proregenerative properties were evaluated	Membrane functionalized with curcumin and aspirin-loaded PLGA nanoparticles	50–85 nm	An antimicrobial effect of the functionalized membrane against *S aureus*, *E coli*, and *E faecalis* was observed. Enhancement of the osteogenic potential at both transcriptional and translational levels. After 28 d, the lesion was completely filled with new bone, whereas the area covered by the commercial membrane remained empty
Pérez-Pacheco et al, 2019[46]	Clinical (6 mo): periodontitis patients received SRP + PLGA/PLA nanoparticles loaded with 50 μg of curcumin or SRP + empty nanoparticles	Curcumin	Not specified	PPD, CAL, and BOP were improved in both groups. A decrease in red complex bacteria was observed in both groups

(continued on next page)

Table 2
(continued)

Study	Type of Study	Active Drug	Size of Particles	Effects
				No difference in terms of GCF cytokine levels were observed between groups
				No additive benefits of a single local application of curcumin
Lecio et al, 2019[47]	Clinical (6 mo): Effect of PLGA nanospheres containing 20% doxycycline on patients with diabetes type II with chronic periodontitis vs PLGA + placebo	Doxycycline	1 μm	Both groups showed clinical improvement in all parameters after treatment
				Doxycycline improved deep pockets, BOP, PPD, and CAL (vs placebo)
				The percentage of sites presenting PPD reduction and CAL gain of ≥2 mm was higher in doxycycline at 3 mo
				Doxycycline induced an increased level of anti-inflammatory IL-10, and a decrease in of IL-8, IFN-γ, IL-6, and IL-17
				A decrease in periodontal pathogen counts
Mahmoud et al, 2019[48]	In vitro: telomerase immortalized gingival keratinocytes In vivo: Measure of alveolar bone destruction in mouse experimental periodontitis Effect of peptide (BAR) derived from *S gordonii* – modified PLGA nanoparticles	BAR (peptide)	333 nm and 312 nm (hydrated)	Less bone loss and IL-17 after treatment
				No significant lysis or apoptosis of telomerase immortalized gingival keratinocytes after treatment relative to untreated cells

Study	Description	Agent	Size	Results
Xue et al, 2019[32]	In vitro: primary human periodontal ligament cells; *E coli* culture. In vivo: Measure of the bone regeneration in the mandible of New Zealand white rabbits. Effect of PLGA nanoparticles, CS nanoparticles, silver nanoparticles and a combination of the 3 were evaluated.		112.4 ± 8.33 nm (PLGA nanoparticles) 180.3 ± 11.2 nm (CS nanoparticles)	Nanoparticles were found to have no significant cytotoxicity and were able to promote human periodontal ligament cells mineralization CS nanoparticles and silver nanoparticles in low concentrations showed antibacterial activity The PLGA nanoparticles and CS nanoparticles complex contributed to cell mineralization and had no cytotoxicity The bone recovery rate of PLGA nanoparticles/CS nanoparticles group was greater than that of PLGA nanoparticles/CS nanoparticles/silver nanoparticles group. Results in both test groups were better than control group
Pereira et al, 2018[49]	In vivo: Evaluation of the effect of metformin hydrochloride-loaded PLGA in a ligature-induced periodontitis model in diabetic rats	Metformin hydrochloride	457.1 ± 48.9 nm	Metformin-loaded PLGA decreased inflammation (IL-1β and tumor necrosis factor -α), and bone loss
Rizzi et al, 2016[50]	In vitro: Human keratinovytes Evaluation of proliferative effects of epiregulin- PLGA nanoparticles on human keratinocytes	Epiregulin	190–370 nm	50:50 PLGA- nanoparticles exhibited the best dental adhesive ability

(continued on next page)

Table 2
(continued)

Study	Type of Study	Active Drug	Size of Particles	Effects
				Epiregulin-loaded nanoparticles increased cell proliferation
Lee et al, 2016[26]	In vitro: human bone marrow-derived osteoblasts; *A actinomycetemcomitans* and *Prevotella nigrescens* culture In vivo: maxillary intrabony defect in dog Evaluation of cytotoxic effect and alkaline phosphatase activity, as well as antibacterial activity and bone regenerative potential of PLGA–lovastatin–chitosan–tetracycline nanoparticles	Lovastatin-chitosan-tetracycline	105–111 nm	PLGA–lovastatin–chitosan–tetracycline nanoparticles showed good biocompatibility, antibacterial activity, and increased alkaline phosphatase activity Increased of new bone formation in defects filled with nanoparticles

Abbreviations: BOP, bleeding on probing; CAL, clinical attachment level; GCF, gingival crevicular fluid; PPD, periodontal pocket depth; SRP, scaling and root planing.

CARBON QUANTUM DOTS

Carbon dots are considered a class of zero-dimensional carbon materials with a size of less than 10 nm, and fluorescence is their intrinsic property.[51] Several processes have been developed to synthesize carbon dots, including chemical ablation, electrochemical carbonization, laser ablation, microwave irradiation, and hydrothermal treatment.[15] To synthesize carbon dots, several carbon sources could be selected. Indeed, bacteria such as *Lactobacillus plantarum*,[52] fruit such as *Cittrus limetta*,[53] and molecules or drugs with antibacterial properties such as metronidazole, tinidazole, and curcumin have been used[15,51,54] (**Table 3**). Interestingly, carbon dots demonstrated ability to be internalized quickly by cells, and, more importantly to decrease biofilm formation, bacterial growth and virulence as observed with *P gingivalis* culture treated with tinidazole carbon dots.[15] In this study, the potential therapeutic effect associated with carbon dots use was also concomitant with an improved penetration within *P gingivalis* biofilm when compared with tinidazole treatment. Owing to their prominent optical properties, carbon dots could also be used to deliver in a site and time-controlled manner an active compound, as observed in vitro in conjunction with the use of photodynamic therapy to activate the delivery of curcumin.[55]

MESOPOROUS SILICA

Mesoporous silica nanoparticles have been proposed as promising drug vehicles because they present large surface area and controlled porosity that allow fine control of the release kinetics of the uploaded drugs. Mesoporous silica attracted interest because they show better loading ability and more sustained and prolonged drug release making them suitable for local delivery of antibiotics and osteoinductive and angiogenic growth factors.[56] Indeed, bioactive glasses have been evaluated extensively to promote bone regeneration in different types of bone defects, such as unloaded critical-sized defects to mechanically loaded, weight-bearing sites with highly favorable outcomes.[57] Several drugs could be loaded in such nanoparticles such as metallic ions (Ag, Cu, etc), but also antibiotics, which could be interesting to decrease the risk of bone infection during healing (**Table 4**). In the context of periodontal regeneration, several studies with different types of mesoporous silica nanoparticles were conducted and demonstrated promising results in terms of biocompatibility and enhancement of the neobone formation such effect being obviously dependent on the drug or active compound loaded.

CLINICAL PERSPECTIVES

Nanomedicine has open new perspectives for periodontitis treatment; as such, developed technologies will contribute to reduce current periodontal treatment limitations. In addition, the modulation of inflammation and the activation of regenerative process through the specific targeting of host cells with controlled and limited dose of pharmacologic agent are required. As described in this review, several strategies are currently developed and, for most of them, induced positive outcomes in terms of antibacterial, anti-inflammatory and prohealing effects. The use of nanoparticles delivery has several advantages. It improves pharmacokinetics and therefore drug efficacy with fewer side effects and toxicity[63] owing mainly, in the context of periodontal treatment, to the local delivery within periodontal lesion. Nanomedicine also targets specific cells to use or activate their machinery. For instance, some therapeutics already target macrophages and monocytes as demonstrated in the context of vascular diseases treatment.[64] Because such cells are also of prime importance in the development of

Table 3
Representative studies evaluating potential use of carbon dots in the context of periodontal treatment

Study	Type of Study	Active Drug	Size and Carbon Source	Effects
Ardekani et al, 2019[54]	In vitro: H413 cells (human oral squamous cell carcinoma)	Metronidazole	1–5 nm; chlorophyll	Chlorophyll was internalized into the cells At a low concentration (0.26 μmol/L), a 72% enhancement of efficacy was observed compared with metronidazole alone
Pourhajibagher et al, 2019[55]	In vitro: primary human gingival fibroblast cells Periodontal pathogens: A actinomycetemcomitans, P gingivalis, and P intermedia	Curcumin	<10 nm; graphene	Graphene–curcumin exhibited no cytotoxicity against human gingival fibroblast cells. Photoexcited graphene–curcumin resulted in a significant reduction in cell viability (93%) and biofilm formation capacity (76%) of periodontal pathogens compared with the control group ($P < .05$).
Liang et al, 2020[15]	In vitro: biofilm (P gingivalis, E coli, S aureus, and Prevotella nigrescens)	Tinidazole Metronidazole	12–20 nm; tinidazole, metronidazole	Inhibitory effect on P gingivalis but not on E coli, S aureus, P nigrescens) Tinidazole could penetrate the biofilms to further effectively inhibit the growth of P gingivalis Tinidazole altered toxicity by inhibiting virulence factors and genes associated in biofilm formation by P gingivalis

Table 4

Representative studies evaluating potential use of mesoporous silica in the context of periodontal treatment

Study	Type of Study	Active Drug	Size	Effects
Pouroutzido et al, 2021[56]	In vitro: Primary human periodontal ligament fibroblast cells Human red blood cells	Moxifloxacin	150–535 nm; mesoporous silica-based nanoparticles (MSNs)	MSNs exhibited no cytotoxicity against human periodontal ligament fibroblast cells. All MSNs co-doped with Ca, Mg, and Sr revealed the formation of hydroxycarbonate apatite on their surface after 10 d of immersion in simulated body fluid and promoted mitochondrial activity and cell proliferation The addition of Mg and Sr up to specific concentrations improved the hemolytic activity and cell proliferation, while maintaining sufficient moxifloxacin loading and sustained release rates
Dexiong et al, 2021[58]	In vitro: BMSCs of Sprague Dawley rat Biofilm (S aureus (ATCC 25923), E coli (ATCC 25922), and P gingivalis (ATCC 33277)	Quaternary ammonium salts and Ag	220–250 nm; Ag@QHMS	Compared with the negative control, the Ag@QHMS groups exhibited better antimicrobial effect Ag@QHMS groups showed a concentration-dependent antibacterial effect on E coli and S aureus that is comparable of the one

(continued on next page)

Table 4
(continued)

Study	Type of Study	Active Drug	Size	Effects
				obtained with the same concentration of pure QHMS
				The inhibition effect of the low concentration of Ag@QHMS on *P gingivalis* is significantly higher than that of the highest concentration of QHMS
				Ag@QHMS promoted calcium deposition and the expression in RUNX2, ALP, OPN, OCN, BSP, and COL-1 gene expression after 2 wk
				Among these markers, the expression of early factors, such as RUNX2 and BSP, did not show large changes, whereas the expression of OPN, ALP ($P < .001$), and COL-1 ($P < .01$) increased considerably because of their accumulation over the entire osteogenesis process
				Ag@QHMS group was the only one to show a statistically significant increase in ALP ($P < .05$) after 1 wk
				Ag@QHMS-containing nanosilver particles has better osteoinductive

| Meifei et al, 2020[59] | In vitro: Mouse fibroblasts (L929 cells) and rat BMSCs
In vivo: rat periodontal defect
Pathogens: E coli, ATCC 25922 and S aureus, ATCC 25923 | Copper (Cu) | 121.45 ± 13.45 nm; Cu@MSNs | activity than pure HMS and QHMS
MSNs and Cu@MSNs exhibited no cytotoxicity against rat BMSCs and L929 cells
Compared with PG-MSNs and pure PG scaffold, PG-Cu@MSNs significantly enhanced ALP expression ($P < .05$), amount of ARS-stained mineralized modules ($P < .01$) and OCN expression
The expression levels of several osteogenic-related genes, including RUNX2, ALP, Col I, and OCN, showed a greater increase in the expression levels of BMSCs cultured on the PG-MSNs and PG-Cu@MSNs scaffolds compared with those on the pure PG scaffolds ($P < .05$)
The incorporation of Cu@MSNs significantly promoted periodontal bone repair in vivo with repaired bone tissue, fully replacing the defect and well-integrating with the surrounding tissues
PG-Cu@MSNs scaffold induced periodontal reattachment connecting the cementum and regenerated bone |

(continued on next page)

Table 4
(continued)

Study	Type of Study	Active Drug	Size	Effects
Lu et al, 2018[60]	In vitro: Human immortalized oral epithelial cells Biofilm (*Streptococcus Mutans* (ATCC 25175) In vivo: mice drug oral administration	Ag and CHX	CHX-loaded, Ag-MSNs@CHX	Initial growth of *S mutans* was time-and dose-dependently delayed with Ag-MSNs@CHX, whereas MSNs only had no effect on the growth of *S mutans* Ag-MSNs@ CHX dose-dependently inhibited the growth of *S. mutans* biofilms Ag-MSNs@CHX group exhibited the strongest biofilm inhibition compared with the other groups Ag-MSNs@CHX could adhere on the bacterial cell surface and induce bacterial cell death accompanied by decoherence of the extracellular matrix. Collectively, these findings demonstrated that Ag-MSNs@CHX efficiently inhibited *S mutans* growth and its biofilm formation Ag-MSNs@CHX significantly decreased the toxicity of CHX in oral epithelial cells and exhibit no abnormal effects on mice after oral administration

| Liu et al, 2018[61] | IL-2/TGF-β and miR-10a | In vitro: Mouse regulatory T cells In vivo: Mouse periodontal disease model | Approximately 100 nm; miR10a-loaded polyplexes 60–90 µm; poly(L-lactic acid) NF-SMS Approximately 300 nm; poly(L-lactic acid)/polyethylene glycol cofunctionalized mesoporous silica nanoparticles Approximately 2 µm; Poly(lactic acid-co-glycolic acid) microspheres | All tested microspheres exhibited no detectable level of cytotoxicity. In vitro after 48 h, IL-2/TGF-β release and miR-10a release facilitated the Treg differentiation, resulting in the generation of functional T regulatory cells from naïve T cells In vivo, combined miR-10a/IL-2/TGF-β release from NF-SMS was significantly more effective than miR-10a release alone or IL-2/TGFβ release alone (also from NF-SMS) in rescuing bone resorption, indicating a synergistic effect between miR-10a and IL-2/TGF-β The gene expression analysis of the isolated gingival tissues showed that the primary cytokines of effector T cells, IL-1β, IL6, IL8, IL17, tumor necrosis factor, IFN-γ and MCP-1 were upregulated in ligature without treatment group, and significantly decreased by the injection of the combined miR-10a/IL2/TGF-β releasing NF-SMS Only the combined miR-10a/IL-2/TGF-β release group could |

(continued on next page)

Table 4
(continued)

Study	Type of Study	Active Drug	Size	Effects
				substantially rescue the bone loss in vivo
Li et al, 2017[62]	In vitro: Primary hGECs	BA and BE	367 ± 94 nm; BA and BE encapsulated in an amine-modified mesoporous silica nanoparticles (Nano-BA and Nano-BE)	BA and Nano-BA exhibited no cytotoxicity against hGECs, Nano-encapsulation greatly enhances the drug delivery rate and prolongs the release of BA and BE up to 216 h Moreover, both Nano-BA and Nano-BE could be internalized by hGECs and retained intracellularly in nanoparticle-free media for at least 24 h Nano-BE pretreatment effectively downregulates the IL-1β–induced expression of IL-6 and IL-8 in hGECs However, pretreatment with Nano-BA was unable to suppress the IL-1β–stimulated expression of IL-6, IL-8 and granulocyte colony stimulating factor

Abbreviations: Ag, silver; Ag-MSNs@CHX, CHX-loaded, Ag-decorated mesoporous silica nanoparticles; Ag@QHMS; quaternary ammonium salts–modified core shell mesoporous silica containing Ag nanoparticles; BA, Baicalin; BE, baicalein; BMSC, bone mesenchymal stem cells; CHX, chlorexidine; Cu@MSNs, copper-loaded mesoporous silica nanoparticles; HGEC, human gingival epithelial cells; MSNs, mesoporous silica-based nanoparticles; NF-SMS, nanofibrous spongy; TGF, transforming growth factor.

periodontal lesion and periodontal healing, such a strategy may be of interest. However, the periodontal application of nanomedicine at the clinical level remains limited. As shown previously, most of the data available are from in vitro or animal studies. Therefore, there is a high need for randomized clinical trials to establish the safety of use and to determine the improvement in terms of periodontal treatment outcomes versus already used techniques with cost, safety, and effectiveness perspectives. Such evaluation could be challenging as specific tests or procedures should be developed as it was demonstrated that some nanoparticles may interfere with common evaluation tests.[65] Nevertheless, the effect of nanoparticles at the lesion site is also determined by the selected scaffold (hydrogel, membranes, hydroxyapatite particles, etc). Therefore, their effects could be associated with the own clinical limitations of the aforementioned scaffolds.

CLINICS CARE POINTS

- Nanomedicine and nanocarriers are developed and used to treat several diseases such as cancer and inflammatory diseases.
- Nanocarriers allow cell-specific targeted delivery of active drugs.
- There is a need for clinical evaluation of nanoparticles use in the context of periodontal treatment and regeneration.
- A cost-effectiveness evaluation should be performed versus already existing biomaterials.

DISCLOSURE

The authors have nothing to disclose.

ACKNOWLEDGMENTS

The authors have no conflicts of interest to declare. The authors thank Prof. C. Serra for the PLGA particle synthesis and imaging. The authors were supported by their own Institutions.

REFERENCES

1. Bosshardt DD, Sculean A. Does periodontal tissue regeneration really work? Periodontol 2000 2009;51:208–19.
2. Harmouche L, Courval A, Mathieu A, et al. Impact of tooth-related factors on photodynamic therapy effectiveness during active periodontal therapy: a 6-months split-mouth randomized clinical trial. Photodiagnosis Photodyn Ther 2019;27:167–72.
3. Eickholz P, Koch R, Kocher T, et al. Clinical benefits of systemic amoxicillin/metronidazole may depend on periodontitis severity and patients' age: an exploratory sub-analysis of the ABPARO trial. J Clin Periodontol 2019;46(4):491–501.
4. Martin-Cabezas R, Davideau J-L, Tenenbaum H, et al. Clinical efficacy of probiotics as an adjunctive therapy to non-surgical periodontal treatment of chronic periodontitis: a systematic review and meta-analysis. J Clin Periodontol 2016; 43(6):520–30.
5. Courval A, Harmouche L, Mathieu A, et al. Impact of molar furcations on photodynamic therapy outcomes: a 6-month split-mouth randomized clinical trial. Int J Environ Res Public Health 2020;17(11):4162.

6. Schwach-Abdellaoui K, Vivien-Castioni N, Gurny R. Local delivery of antimicrobial agents for the treatment of periodontal diseases. Eur J Pharm Biopharm 2000;50(1):83–99.

7. Steinberg D, Friedman M. Sustained-release delivery of antimicrobial drugs for the treatment of periodontal diseases: fantasy or already reality? Periodontol 2000 2020;84(1):176–87.

8. Mali S. Nanomedicine–next generation technology revolutionizing medical practice. J Maxillofac Oral Surg 2013;12(1):1–2.

9. He H, Liu L, Morin EE, et al. Survey of clinical translation of cancer nanomedicines-lessons learned from successes and failures. Acc Chem Res 2019;52(9):2445–61.

10. Yu Z, Reynaud F, Lorscheider M, et al. Nanomedicines for the delivery of glucocorticoids and nucleic acids as potential alternatives in the treatment of rheumatoid arthritis. Interdiscip Rev Nanomed Nanobiotechnol 2020;12(5):e1630.

11. Bosshardt DD. The periodontal pocket: pathogenesis, histopathology and consequences. Periodontol 2000 2018;76(1):43–50.

12. Suárez LJ, Garzón H, Arboleda S, et al. Oral dysbiosis and autoimmunity: from local periodontal responses to an imbalanced systemic immunity. a review. Front Immunol 2020;11:591255.

13. Vitkov L, Minnich B, Knopf J, et al. NETs are double-edged swords with the potential to aggravate or resolve periodontal inflammation. Cells 2020;9(12):2614.

14. Cafferata EA, Alvarez C, Diaz KT, et al. Multifunctional nanocarriers for the treatment of periodontitis: immunomodulatory, antimicrobial, and regenerative strategies. Oral Dis 2019;25(8):1866–78.

15. Liang G, Shi H, Qi Y, et al. Specific anti-biofilm activity of carbon quantum dots by destroying P. gingivalis biofilm related genes. Int J Nanomedicine 2020;15: 5473–89.

16. Aguilar A, Zein N, Harmouch E, et al. Application of chitosan in bone and dental engineering. Mol 2019;24(16):3009.

17. Kumari S, Tiyyagura HR, Pottathara YB, et al. Surface functionalization of chitosan as a coating material for orthopaedic applications: a comprehensive review. Carbohydr Polym 2021;255:117487.

18. Hu Z, Zhang D-Y, Lu S-T, et al. Chitosan-based composite materials for prospective hemostatic applications. Mar Drugs 2018;16(8):273.

19. Saini S, Dhiman A, Nanda S. Immunomodulatory properties of chitosan: impact on wound healing and tissue repair. Endocr Metab Immune Disord Drug Targets 2020;20(10):1611–23.

20. Arancibia R, Maturana C, Silva D, et al. Effects of chitosan particles in periodontal pathogens and gingival fibroblasts. J Dent Res 2013;92(8):740–5.

21. Hu Y, Chen Y, Lin L, et al. Studies on antimicrobial peptide-loaded nanomaterial for root caries restorations to inhibit periodontitis related pathogens in periodontitis care. J Microencapsul 2021;38:89–99.

22. Barreras US, Méndez FT, Martínez REM, et al. Chitosan nanoparticles enhance the antibacterial activity of chlorhexidine in collagen membranes used for periapical guided tissue regeneration. Mater Sci Eng C Mater Biol Appl 2016;58: 1182–7.

23. Martin V, Ribeiro IAC, Alves MM, et al. Understanding intracellular trafficking and anti-inflammatory effects of minocycline chitosan-nanoparticles in human gingival fibroblasts for periodontal disease treatment. Int J Pharm 2019;572:118821.

24. Eap S, Ferrand A, Schiavi J, et al. Collagen implants equipped with 'fish scale'-like nanoreservoirs of growth factors for bone regeneration. Nanomed 2014; 9(8):1253–61.

25. Ferrand A, Eap S, Richert L, et al. Osteogenetic properties of electrospun nanofibrous PCL scaffolds equipped with chitosan-based nanoreservoirs of growth factors. Macromol Biosci 2014;14(1):45–55.

26. Lee B-S, Lee C-C, Wang Y-P, et al. Controlled-release of tetracycline and lovastatin by poly(D,L-lactide-co-glycolide acid)-chitosan nanoparticles enhances periodontal regeneration in dogs. Int J Nanomedicine 2016;11:285–97.

27. Petit C, Batool F, Stutz C, et al. Development of a thermosensitive statin loaded chitosan-based hydrogel promoting bone healing. Int J Pharm 2020;586:119534.

28. Stutz C, Strub M, Clauss F, et al. A new polycaprolactone-based biomembrane functionalized with BMP-2 and Stem cells improves maxillary bone regeneration. Nanomaterials (Basel) 2020;10(9):1774.

29. Soe HMSH, Luckanagul JA, Pavasant P, et al. Development of in situ gel containing asiaticoside/cyclodextrin complexes. Evaluation in culture human periodontal ligament cells (HPLDCs). Int J Pharm 2020;586:119589.

30. Xu S, Zhou Q, Jiang Z, et al. The effect of doxycycline-containing chitosan/carboxymethyl chitosan nanoparticles on NLRP3 inflammasome in periodontal disease. Carbohydr Polym 2020;237:116163.

31. Aminu N, Chan S-Y, Yam M-F, et al. A dual-action chitosan-based nanogel system of triclosan and flurbiprofen for localised treatment of periodontitis. Int J Pharm 2019;570:118659.

32. Preparation and biological characterization of the mixture of poly(lactic-co-glycolic acid)/chitosan/Ag nanoparticles for periodontal tissue engineering. Int J Nanomed 2019;14:483–98.

33. Hu F, Zhou Z, Xu Q, et al. A novel pH-responsive quaternary ammonium chitosan-liposome nanoparticles for periodontal treatment. Int J Biol Macromol 2019;129:1113–9.

34. He Y, Jin Y, Wang X, et al. An antimicrobial peptide-loaded gelatin/chitosan nanofibrous membrane fabricated by sequential layer-by-layer electrospinning and electrospraying techniques. Nanomaterials (Basel) 2018;8(5):327.

35. Guarino V, Cruz-Maya I, Altobelli R, et al. Electrospun polycaprolactone nanofibres decorated by drug loaded chitosan nano-reservoirs for antibacterial treatments. Nanotechnology 2017;28(50):505103.

36. Lin J-H, Feng F, Yu M-C, et al. Modulation of periodontitis progression using pH-responsive nanosphere encapsulating metronidazole or N-phenacylthialzolium bromide. J Periodontal Res 2018;53(1):22–8.

37. Li H, Ji Q, Chen X, et al. Accelerated bony defect healing based on chitosan thermosensitive hydrogel scaffolds embedded with chitosan nanoparticles for the delivery of BMP2 plasmid DNA. J Biomed Mater Res A 2017;105(1):265–73.

38. Li D-D, Pan J-F, Ji Q-X, et al. Characterization and cytocompatibility of thermosensitive hydrogel embedded with chitosan nanoparticles for delivery of bone morphogenetic protein-2 plasmid DNA. J Mater Sci Mater Med 2016;27(8):134.

39. Kumari A, Yadav SK, Yadav SC. Biodegradable polymeric nanoparticles based drug delivery systems. Colloids Surf B Biointerfaces 2010;75(1):1–18.

40. Sun X, Xu C, Wu G, et al. Poly(lactic-co-glycolic acid): applications and future prospects for periodontal tissue regeneration. Polymers (Basel) 2017;9(6):189.

41. Chang P-C, Tai W-C, Luo H-T, et al. Core-shell poly-(D,l-lactide-co-glycolide)-chitosan nanospheres with simvastatin-doxycycline for periodontal and osseous repair. Int J Biol Macromol 2020;158:627–35.

42. de Freitas LM, Calixto GMF, Chorilli M, et al. Polymeric nanoparticle-based photo-dynamic therapy for chronic periodontitis in vivo. Int J Mol Sci 2016;17(5):769.

43. Klepac-Ceraj V, Patel N, Song X, et al. Photodynamic effects of methylene blue-loaded polymeric nanoparticles on dental plaque bacteria. Lasers Surg Med 2011;43(7):600–6.

44. Beg S, Dhiman S, Sharma T, et al. Stimuli responsive in situ gelling systems loaded with PLGA nanoparticles of moxifloxacin hydrochloride for effective treatment of periodontitis. AAPS PharmSciTech 2020;21(3):76.

45. Ghavimi MA, Bani Shahabadi A, Jarolmasjed S, et al. Nanofibrous asymmetric collagen/curcumin membrane containing aspirin-loaded PLGA nanoparticles for guided bone regeneration. Sci Rep 2020;10(1):18200.

46. Pérez-Pacheco CG, Fernandes NAR, Primo FL, et al. Local application of curcumin-loaded nanoparticles as an adjunct to scaling and root planing in periodontitis: Randomized, placebo-controlled, double-blind split-mouth clinical trial. Clin Oral Investig 2021;25(5):3217–27.

47. Lecio G, Ribeiro FV, Pimentel SP, et al. Novel 20% doxycycline-loaded PLGA nanospheres as adjunctive therapy in chronic periodontitis in type-2 diabetics: randomized clinical, immune and microbiological trial. Clin Oral Investig 2020; 24(3):1269–79.

48. Mahmoud MY, Steinbach-Rankins JM, Demuth DR. Functional assessment of peptide-modified PLGA nanoparticles against oral biofilms in a murine model of periodontitis. J Control Release 2019;297:3–13.

49. Pereira ASBF, Brito GAC, Lima MLS, et al. Metformin hydrochloride-loaded PLGA nanoparticle in periodontal disease experimental model using diabetic rats. Int J Mol Sci 2018;19(11):3488.

50. Rizzi M, Migliario M, Rocchetti V, et al. Epiregulin-loaded PLGA nanoparticles increase human keratinocytes proliferation: preliminary data. Eur Rev Med Pharmacol Sci 2016;20(12):2484–90.

51. Liu J, Lu S, Tang Q, et al. One-step hydrothermal synthesis of photoluminescent carbon nanodots with selective antibacterial activity against Porphyromonas gingivalis. Nanoscale 2017;9(21):7135–42.

52. Lin F, Li C, Chen Z. Bacteria-derived carbon dots inhibit biofilm formation of Escherichia coli without affecting cell growth. Front Microbiol 2018;9:259.

53. Shaikh AF, Tamboli MS, Patil RH, et al. Bioinspired carbon quantum dots: an anti-biofilm agents. J Nanosci Nanotechnol 2019;19(4):2339–45.

54. Ardekani SM, Dehghani A, Ye P, et al. Conjugated carbon quantum dots: Potent nano-antibiotic for intracellular pathogens. J Colloid Interf Sci 2019;552:378–87.

55. Pourhajibagher M, Parker S, Chiniforush N, et al. Photoexcitation triggering via semiconductor graphene quantum dots by photochemical doping with curcumin versus perio-pathogens mixed biofilms. Photodiagnosis Photodyn Ther 2019;28: 125–31.

56. Pouroutzidou GK, Liverani L, Theocharidou A, et al. Synthesis and characterization of mesoporous Mg- and Sr-doped nanoparticles for moxifloxacin drug delivery in promising tissue engineering applications. Int J Mol Sci 2021;22(2).

57. Liang W, Wu X, Dong Y, et al. In vivo behavior of bioactive glass-based composites in animal models for bone regeneration. Biomater Sci 2021;9(6):1924–44.

58. Li D, Qiu Y, Zhang S, et al. A multifunctional antibacterial and osteogenic nanomedicine: QAS-modified core-shell mesoporous silica containing Ag nanoparticles. Biomed Res Int 2020;2020:4567049.

59. Lian M, Han Y, Sun B, et al. A multifunctional electrowritten bi-layered scaffold for guided bone regeneration. Acta Biomater 2020;118:83–99.

60. Lu M-M, Ge Y, Qiu J, et al. Redox/pH dual-controlled release of chlorhexidine and silver ions from biodegradable mesoporous silica nanoparticles against oral biofilms. Int J Nanomedicine 2018;13:7697–709.
61. Liu Z, Chen X, Zhang Z, et al. Nanofibrous spongy microspheres to distinctly release miRNA and growth factors to enrich regulatory T cells and rescue periodontal bone loss. ACS Nano 2018;12(10):9785–99.
62. Li X, Luo W, Ng TW, et al. Nanoparticle-encapsulated baicalein markedly modulates pro-inflammatory response in gingival epithelial cells. Nanoscale 2017; 9(35):12897–907.
63. Igarashi E. Factors affecting toxicity and efficacy of polymeric nanomedicines. Toxicol Appl Pharmacol 2008;229(1):121–34.
64. Katsuki S, Koga J-I, Matoba T, et al. Nanoparticle-mediated delivery of pitavastatin to monocytes/macrophages inhibits angiotensin ii-induced abdominal aortic aneurysm formation in Apoe -/- mice. J Atheroscler Thromb 2021. https://doi.org/10.5551/jat.54379.
65. McMillan J, Batrakova E, Gendelman HE. Cell delivery of therapeutic nanoparticles. Prog Mol Biol Transl Sci 2011;104:563–601.

Biomarkers and Periodontal Regenerative Approaches

Ulvi Kahraman Gürsoy, DDS, PhD*, Mervi Gürsoy, DDS, PhD, Eija Könönen, DDS, PhD

KEYWORDS

- Alveolar bone • Biomarker • Periodontal ligament • Regeneration

KEY POINTS

- Simple and reliable methods that can observe periodontal tissue regeneration will bring significant advantages to dental clinicians.
- In medicine, various serum proteins have been studied as potential biomarkers of osteoblast or osteoclast activities.
- Available data are not enough to propose the use of any specific biomarker in determination of periodontal regeneration.
- Bone alkaline phosphatase and osteocalcin are potential biomarker candidates to predict and follow the success of periodontal regeneration after treatment.

INTRODUCTION

Periodontal disease is of infectious origin and inflammatory character, where chronic and uncontrolled immune responses initiate the process that leads to the destruction of tooth-supporting tissues and, if untreated, eventually to tooth loss. During the disease process, the balance between removal and regeneration of periodontal tissue components is disrupted: new tissue formation activated by keratinocytes, fibroblasts, and osteoblasts is suppressed, whereas tissue degradation activated by neutrophils, macrophages, and osteoclasts is stimulated. The integrity of the junctional epithelium, periodontal ligament, and alveolar bone is broken in some degrees, depending on the stage of periodontitis.[1]

Periodontal tissue damage around the affected teeth can be measured by using clinical (probing pocket depth [PPD], clinical attachment level [CAL]) or radiographic (alveolar bone loss) indices. In most cases, it is possible to prevent the disease progression using nonsurgical and surgical periodontal therapies; however, replacing the damaged periodontal tissues with the physically and functionally similar structures (ie, regeneration) remains challenging.[2] Periodontal regeneration is the ultimate goal of

Department of Periodontology, Institute of Dentistry, University of Turku, Lemminkäisenkatu 2, 20520 Turku, Finland
* Corresponding author.
E-mail address: ulvi.gursoy@utu.fi

Dent Clin N Am 66 (2022) 157–167
https://doi.org/10.1016/j.cden.2021.06.006
0011-8532/22/© 2021 Elsevier Inc. All rights reserved.

dental.theclinics.com

periodontal therapy, and the anatomic form, localization, and extent of the periodontal defect are local determinants of periodontal treatment to be applied.[3] In general, residual pockets with 2- to 3-wall intrabony defects are accepted as the most favorable cases for periodontal regeneration, because these defects can successfully regenerate after minimally invasive surgical and minimally invasive nonsurgical treatments, without the need of complicated surgical procedures.[4] Nevertheless, various bone regenerative substitutes and biological agents with osteoinductive or osteoconductive properties are widely used in periodontal practice to get new bone around periodontitis-affected teeth.[5]

Randomized controlled studies have documented the potential of various regenerative therapies to achieve periodontal regeneration in periodontal defects; however, the predictability of treatment success or failure is still a challenge. The outcome of the treatment can differ between 2 identical defects because the regeneration is influenced by multiple factors related to patient, surgical approach, and defect site. As the periodontal regenerative treatments are expensive and time-consuming, clinical use of biological markers that indicate the success or failure of the treatment at its early phases would be beneficial.

Technological advancements and breakthroughs during the last 3 decades have improved our quality of life significantly. Moreover, these advancements have influenced oral sciences, because nowadays it is possible to quantify previously undetectable host or bacterial proteins from patient samples as well as to relate their levels to disease diagnosis, prognosis, or treatment response.[6]

This narrative review aims to discuss periodontal regeneration, that is, regeneration of alveolar bone and periodontal ligament, from biomarker research perspective and to present the available evidence on the use of regeneration-related biomarkers in periodontology. Biomarkers of periodontal wound healing and pocket depth reduction are not included in this review, because they do not necessarily represent regeneration.

BIOLOGICAL MARKERS: BIOMARKERS

A biomarker is "a characteristic that is objectively measured and evaluated as an indicator of normal biological processes, pathogenic processes, or pharmacologic responses to a therapeutic intervention" as defined by the working group of the National Institutes of Health Director's Initiative on Biomarkers and Surrogate Endpoints.[7] In general, biomarkers are applied to clinical study designs to get fast and reliable information on an objectively defined clinical outcome (clinical endpoint). In such study designs, a well-validated biomarker (ie, with high sensitivity, specificity, and reproducibility), which has either a causal or mechanistic association with the disease pathogenesis or therapeutic intervention, functions as a surrogate end point to predict the clinical end point. Overall, biomarkers are used to (1) diagnose a disease, (2) stage or classify the extension of the disease, (3) follow the disease prognosis, and (4) predict or monitor the treatment outcome.[7]

BIOMARKER RESEARCH IN PERIODONTOLOGY

In periodontology, searches for quantifiable and easy-to-detect biomarkers from noninvasively collected biological samples (saliva, oral rinse, gingival crevicular fluid) are not new. Indeed, for decades, researchers have looked for biomarkers to detect disease, disease initiation, disease progression, successful treatment outcomes, and periodontal regeneration[8,9] (Table 1). Most biomarker studies in periodontology have been performed either to discriminate patients with periodontitis from

Table 1
Applied biomarker types related to clinical applications in periodontology

Marker types	Potential applications
Genetic markers (eg, interleukin-1, mannose-binding lectin genotypes)	• Indicating a potential risk to develop periodontitis • Estimating healing response after periodontal treatment
Infectious and inflammatory markers (eg, *Porphyromonas gingivalis* and its gingipain, interleukin-1β, interleukin-17, tumor necrosis factor-α)	• Early detection of periodontitis • Estimating the prognosis of periodontitis • Estimating healing response after periodontal treatment
Wound healing markers (eg, keratinocyte growth factor, basic fibroblast growth factor)	• Estimating soft tissue healing response after periodontal treatment
Regeneration markers (eg, alkaline phosphatase, osteocalcin)	• Estimating response to periodontal regenerative treatment

periodontally healthy individuals (at the population level) or to detect disease activity in periodontal pockets (at the site level).[10] It is indeed understandable that the "susceptibility to develop periodontitis," "initiation of periodontitis," or "periodontal regeneration" has been rarely applied as periodontal end points, because these outcomes require longitudinal studies. To validate a biomarker's sensitivity and specificity to detect "susceptibility to develop periodontitis" or "initiation of periodontitis," a large number of individuals need to be followed over years and preferably must not be treated when study participants develop gingivitis. This type of study design will be neither ethically nor financially possible.

Until now various host and bacterial proteins, including matrix metalloproteinase (MMP)-8, interleukin (IL)-1β, and *Porphyromonas gingivalis* or its gingipains, have been demonstrated to be successful in diagnosing periodontitis and to predict the healing response after periodontal treatment.[9,11,12]

BIOMARKERS OF PERIODONTAL REGENERATION: OBSTACLES

Research targeted to define a periodontal regeneration biomarker has some obstacles. First, as a general rule in biomarker studies, the primary clinical end point needs to be precisely defined and measured objectively. To give an example, when "periodontitis" is taken as a clinical end point, it is defined precisely as "periodontal tissue destruction due to inflammation as a primary feature, with a threshold of interproximal, clinical attachment loss of ≥4 mm at ≥2 non-adjacent teeth."[13] Here, the levels of inflammation and interproximal clinical attachment loss can be measured objectively. On the contrary, periodontal regeneration, that is, formation of new bone and periodontal attachment, does not have a precise and globally accepted clinical definition. Moreover, gold-standard detection methods of periodontal regeneration are either (1) determination of new bone formation by surgical reopening of the defect area, which is highly invasive and costly, or (2) radiographic determination of bone gain, which can only detect already matured bone (ie, cannot reveal early bone formation).[14]

Another limitation in determining periodontal regeneration biomarkers is related to the biology of new tissue formation. Periodontitis is a degenerative disease regulated by inflammation, where levels of proinflammatory cytokines (eg, IL-1β, IL-6, IL-8, IL-17, tumor necrosis factor [TNF]-α), bacterial and host proteases (eg, *P gingivalis* gingipains, MMPs), and tissue degradation end products (eg, cross-linked carboxy terminal telopeptide of type I collagen) are highly elevated in active phase of the disease.[15] These biomarkers can be easily detected in gingival crevicular fluid or in saliva with current laboratory methods. Periodontal regeneration, however, is a slow and long-term process, which does not lead to a rapid synthesis of signaling molecules (**Fig. 1**). Moreover, extracellular levels of new tissue formation-inducing signaling molecules during regeneration do not increase as significantly as those of proinflammatory cytokines or proteolytic enzymes during active periodontitis.[16] Therefore, measuring alveolar bone regeneration-related marker levels in oral biological fluids, especially in saliva and oral rinse, with current methodological techniques is troublesome.

BIOMARKERS OF PERIODONTAL REGENERATION: POTENTIAL TARGETS

The periosteum, periodontal ligament, and alveolar bone walls act as reservoirs for the cells that take part in periodontal regeneration. Growth and differentiation factors are the major regulators of cellular behaviors. Among them, bone morphogenic proteins, growth differentiation factors, platelet-derived growth factor, fibroblast growth factor

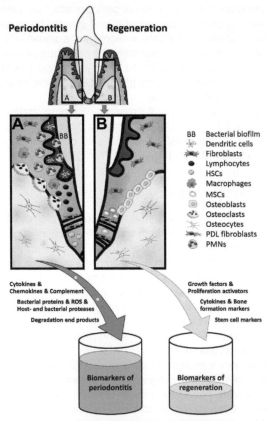

Fig. 1. Cellular and molecular components of periodontitis (*A*) and periodontal regeneration (*B*). HSCs, hematopoietic stem cells; MSCs, mesenchymal stem cells; PDL, periodontal ligament; PMN, polymorphonuclear leukocyte.

(FGF), insulin-like growth factor (IGF), transforming growth factor (TGF)-β, and regeneration signaling pathways (Wnt, FGF, TGF-β signaling) have been extensively studied.[17]

Bone is a dynamic tissue and undergoes continuous remodeling (resorption, reversal, formation) throughout the life.[18] Both remodeling and regeneration of alveolar bone depend on systemic and local factors and may show significant variations between individuals, teeth, and periodontal sites. Understanding the mechanical and biological properties of bone tissue allows researchers to develop new surgical techniques and bioactive molecules that may support regeneration; yet, predicting the tissue response and the rate of regeneration is still a challenge.[5]

During a physiologic remodeling process, the resorption of old bone by osteoclasts and formation of new bone by osteoblasts are in a delicate balance. Although osteoclasts are not included in bone formation, coupling of osteoclasts to osteoblast function is required for the maturation of new bone.[19] The main events that regulate new bone formation include the mesenchymal stem cell recruitment, nonmineralized matrix deposition, osteoblast differentiation, and mineralization. Among signaling pathways, the Wnt pathway was related to osteogenic gene expression in alveolar bone in mice.[20] mRNA expressions of alkaline phosphatase (ALP), osteoprotegerin, osteopontin, osteocalcin, and bone sialoprotein have been detected in newly formed alveolar bone.[21] Although growth factors are responsible for the recruitment, migration, differentiation, and proliferation of regenerative cells and bone formation,[22] studies investigating the associations between serum growth factor levels and bone turnover have yielded conflicting results.[23] For example, IGF levels in serum were found to be associated[24] or not associated[25] with new bone formation.

In medicine, bone alkaline protease (BALP), total osteocalcin, and procollagen type I N-terminal propeptide (P1NP) levels in serum are used as sensitive and reliable markers of new bone formation.[17]

ALP is an enzyme that is produced mainly by the liver, bones, intestines, and kidneys. Serum levels of ALP vary by gender, age, pregnancy, and blood type, and its unusual levels refer to diseases of the liver (primary biliary cirrhosis) or bone (rickets, osteomalacia).[26] BALP is an osteoblast enzyme and functions in new bone mineralization. In a systemically healthy adult, bones produce about 50% of the ALP present in serum.[17] Various laboratory methods, including enzyme immunoassays and immunoradiometric assays, have been applied to specifically detect BALP levels and relate them to new bone formation levels.[26] Immunohistochemical studies on rats and humans have demonstrated a strong ALP positivity in newly formed alveolar bone.[21,27] Elevated numbers of ALP-positive cells were also detected in relation to the inhibition of alveolar bone loss in periodontitis-induced rats.[28] In orthodontic treatment studies[29,30] and in immunohistochemical studies using human and animal models,[31] BALP activity levels correlate with new bone formation. BALP can be measured by electrophoresis, immunoassays, and high-performance liquid chromatography-based methods. Although immunoassays produce the most reproducible and precise results, the cross-reactivity of BALP antibodies with the liver isoform, ALP, is the major limitation of immunoassay use.[32]

Osteocalcin is a small matrix protein, which is synthesized by mature osteoblasts, odontoblasts, and chondrocytes. The main functions of osteocalcin are connected to bone mineralization and calcium ion homeostasis.[33] In patients with osteoporosis, osteocalcin has been effectively used for the determination of osteoblast function and drug-induced bone formation.[34] Elevated numbers of osteocalcin-positive cells after taxifolin treatment were immunohistochemically demonstrated in an experimental periodontitis model in rats.[28] Various methods, including enzyme-linked immunosorbent assay (ELISA), bead-based immunoassay, and chemiluminesence immunoassays, are used in detecting osteocalcin; however, the results may vary between different methods due to the heterogeneity of osteocalcin in the circulation. Furthermore, the reproducibility of osteocalcin level measurements is problematic, because osteocalcin is rapidly degraded into fragments in the circulation and has a short half-life (~5 min).[32] Moreover, increased osteocalcin levels in can be detected in the serum of individuals with renal failure, because osteocalcin is degraded by the kidneys.[17]

P1NP and procollagen type 1 C-terminal propeptide (P1CP) are by-products of the collagen synthesis and thus biomarkers of collagen deposition. Type I collagen forms 90% of the organic bone matrix. During the collagen synthesis, P1NP and P1CP are released into the intracellular space in trimeric structures and can be detected in serum.[17] The unstable trimeric form degrades into stable monomers and fragments that may affect its detectability. Radioimmunoassay and ELISA are methods developed to detect serum P1NP levels.[35]

BIOMARKERS OF PERIODONTAL REGENERATION: EVIDENCE

Evidence on the use of biomarkers to predict periodontal regeneration is highly limited. In the literature, there are numerous studies that relate biomarker levels to posttreatment clinical outcomes. However, the selected clinical end points among the studies vary significantly. The most commonly used clinical end points are (1) inhibited disease progression (elimination of clinical signs of inflammation),[12] (2) reduced pocket depths (formation of long junctional epithelium),[36,37] or (3) periodontal regeneration (periodontal attachment and alveolar bone gain).[38] Notably, neither decreased bleeding on probing nor reduced PPDs indicate periodontal regeneration, thus these studies were not included in this section. Also, studies using salivary biomarkers[39–41] were not included, because they cannot be related to site-specific changes. Hereby, we present the available evidence collected from clinical studies where both periodontal regeneration (CAL gain or radiographic evidence of new bone formation) was taken as a clinical end point and the biomarker and periodontal regeneration levels were quantified from the same tooth site.

No reports on biomarkers in relation to new bone formation were found. In 4 studies, biomarker levels were quantified in gingival crevicular fluid and related to CAL gain[29,42–44] (**Table 2**). Perinetti and coworkers[29] showed a correlation between the ALP activity in gingival crevicular fluid and CAL gain, whereas Pellegrini and coworkers[42] suggested that elevated endothelial growth factor levels in gingival crevicular fluid at baseline indicate posttreatment CAL gain.

In all these 4 studies, CAL was defined as "probing pocket depth in mm + gingival recession in mm." Unfortunately, none of these studies demonstrated any radiographic evidence of periodontal regeneration as part of the clinical outcome. The study by Pellegrini and colleagues[42] (2017) reported that standardized intraoral radiographs of the defects were obtained at baseline and 6 months after periodontal surgery; however, clinical outcome was evaluated only in terms of percentage pocket depth reduction and percentage CAL gain.

DISCUSSION

Regenerative approaches are widely used in periodontology, yet their clinical outcomes vary significantly and are not always predictable. Therefore, there is a need of biomarkers that can real-time monitor biological changes on periodontal tissues to predict the outcome of regenerative treatment. It is evident that the current available

Table 2
Human clinical studies with evidence on the validity of biomarkers in relation to periodontal regeneration

Study	n	Treatment	Clinical end point	End point evaluation	Biomarkers of regeneration	Sample fluid	Findings
Perinetti et al.,[29] 2008	16	SRP	CAL gain	Probing	ALP activity	GCF	Correlation between ALP and CAL gain levels
Pellegrini et al.,[42] 2017	25	GTR & OFD	CAL gain	Probing	BMP-7, EGF, FGF-2, OPG, TGF-β1, VEGF	GCF	Elevated baseline EGF levels may predict CAL gain
Taiete et al.,[44] 2019	24	SRP	CAL gain	Probing	IL-10	GCF	No association with CAL gain
Rakmanee et al.,[43] 2019	18	GTR & AF	CAL gain	Probing	BMP-2, OPG, bFGF, ANG-1, TIMP-1	GCF	No association with CAL gain

Abbreviations: ANG-1, angiopoietin-1; BMP, bone morphogenetic protein; EGF, endothelial growth factor; GCF, gingival crevicular fluid; GTR, guided tissue regeneration; OFD, open flap debridement; OPG, osteoprotegerin; SRP, scaling and root planning; TIMP-1, tissue inhibitor of matrix metalloproteinase-1; VEGF, vascular endothelial growth factor.

data are not enough to propose the use of a specific biomarker in the determination of periodontal regeneration. The vast number of studies reporting on biomarker levels in gingival crevicular fluid, saliva, or oral rinse samples during healing of periodontal defects does not produce evidence of posttreatment tissue regeneration.[3,45]

Radiographic evidence on new bone formation was not implemented in any of the biomarker studies, making the selected end point, CAL gain, questionable. The observed posttreatment CAL gain could be explained by the formation of a long junctional epithelium seen as a reduced pocket depth, with only a minimum amount of periodontal regeneration.[46] Moreover, endogenous (eg, age, gender, and ethnicity) and exogenous (eg, circadian rhythm, exercise, seasonal variations) factors that have an effect on bone regeneration[32] need to be considered as confounding factors.

Taken together, owing to limitations of scientific evidence, only BALP and osteocalcin seem to be the 2 potential biomarkers of periodontal tissue regeneration so far. To define the most reliable biomarkers of periodontal regeneration, there is need of follow-up studies in which the clinical or radiographic evidence of new periodontal attachment and alveolar bone formation was documented in relation to selected biomarker candidates of regeneration.

CLINICS CARE POINTS

- Periodontal therapy aims to eliminate the infection and regenerate the lost tissues.
- Various surgical techniques and biomaterials are used to regain the lost periodontal tissues; however, their outcome is not always predictable.
- Real-time monitoring of biomarkers to follow biological changes after regenerative treatment will guide clinicians to predict clinical outcomes precisely.

DISCLOSURE

The authors have nothing to disclose.

REFERENCES

1. Könönen E, Gürsoy M, Gursoy UK. Periodontitis: A multifaceted disease of tooth-supporting tissues. J Clin Med 2019;8:1135.
2. Bartold PM, Gronthos S, Ivanovski S, et al. Tissue engineered periodontal products. J Periodontal Res 2016;51:1–15.
3. Koidou VP, Chatzopoulos GS, Tomas I, et al. Expression of gingival crevicular fluid markers during early and late healing of intrabony defects after surgical treatment: A systematic review. Clin Oral Investig 2020;24:487–502.
4. Barbato L, Selvaggi F, Kalemaj Z, et al. Clinical efficacy of minimally invasive surgical (MIS) and non-surgical (MINST) treatments of periodontal intra-bony defect. A systematic review and network meta-analysis of RCT's. Clin Oral Investig 2020;24:1125–35.
5. Borciani G, Montalbano G, Baldini N, et al. Co-culture systems of osteoblasts and osteoclasts: Simulating in vitro bone remodeling in regenerative approaches. Acta Biomater 2020;108:22–45.
6. Bernotiene E, Bagdonas E, Kirdaite G, et al. Emerging technologies and platforms for the immunodetection of multiple biochemical markers in osteoarthritis research and therapy. Front Med (Lausanne) 2020;7:572977.

7. Biomarkers Definitions Working Group. Biomarkers and surrogate endpoints: Preferred definitions and conceptual framework. Clin Pharmacol Ther 2001;69: 89–95.

8. Giannobile WV. Salivary diagnostics for periodontal diseases. J Am Dent Assoc 2012;143:6S–11S.

9. Steigmann L, Maekawa S, Sima C, et al. Biosensor and lab-on-a-chip biomarker-identifying technologies for oral and periodontal diseases. Front Pharmacol 2020; 11:588480.

10. Arias-Bujanda N, Regueira-Iglesias A, Balsa-Castro C, et al. Accuracy of single molecular biomarkers in saliva for the diagnosis of periodontitis: A systematic review and meta-analysis. J Clin Periodontol 2020;47:2–18.

11. Gursoy UK, Könönen E, Pussinen PJ, et al. Use of host- and bacteria-derived salivary markers in detection of periodontitis: A cumulative approach. Dis Markers 2011;30:299–305.

12. Gürsoy UK, Fteita D, Bikker FJ, et al. Elevated baseline salivary protease activity may predict the steadiness of gingival inflammation during periodontal healing: A 12-week follow-up study on adults. Pathogens 2020;9:751.

13. Papapanou PN, Sanz M, Buduneli N, et al. Periodontitis: Consensus report of workgroup 2 of the 2017 world workshop on the classification of periodontal and peri-implant diseases and conditions. J Clin Periodontol 2018;45:162–70.

14. Yun JH, Hwang SJ, Kim CS, et al. The correlation between the bone probing, radiographic and histometric measurements of bone level after regenerative surgery. J Periodontal Res 2005;40:453–60.

15. Kurgan S, Kantarci A. Molecular basis for immunohistochemical and inflammatory changes during progression of gingivitis to periodontitis. Periodontol 2000 2018;76:51–67.

16. Carmagnola D, Pellegrini G, Dellavia C, et al. Tissue engineering in periodontology: Biological mediators for periodontal regeneration. Int J Artif Organs 2019;42: 241–57.

17. Giannobile WV, Berglundh T, Al-Nawas B, et al. Biological factors involved in alveolar bone regeneration: Consensus report of working group 1 of the 15th European workshop on periodontology on bone regeneration. J Clin Periodontol 2019;46(Suppl 21):6–11.

18. Szulc P. Bone turnover: Biology and assessment tools. Best Pract Res Clin Endocrinol Metab 2018;32:725–38.

19. Weivoda MM, Chew CK, Monroe DG, et al. Identification of osteoclast-osteoblast coupling factors in humans reveals links between bone and energy metabolism. Nat Commun 2020;11:87.

20. Lim WH, Liu B, Mah SJ, et al. Alveolar bone turnover and periodontal ligament width are controlled by Wnt. J Periodontol 2015;86:319–26.

21. Lima LL, Gonçalves PF, Sallum EA, et al. Guided tissue regeneration may modulate gene expression in periodontal intrabony defects: A human study. J Periodontal Res 2008;43:459–64.

22. Zarei F, Soleimaninejad M. Role of growth factors and biomaterials in wound healing. Artif Cells Nanomed Biotechnol 2018;46(Suppl 1):906–11.

23. Niemann I, Hannemann A, Nauck M, et al. The association between insulin-like growth factor I and bone turnover markers in the general adult population. Bone 2013;56:184–90.

24. Fatayerji D, Eastell R. Age-related changes in bone turnover in men. J Bone Miner Res 1999;14:1203–10.

25. Gurlek A, Gedik O. Endogenous sex steroid, GH and IGF-I levels in normal elderly men: Relationships with bone mineral density and markers of bone turnover. J Endocrinol Invest 2001;24:408–14.

26. Kuo TR, Chen CH. Bone biomarker for the clinical assessment of osteoporosis: Recent developments and future perspectives. Biomarker Res 2017;5:18.

27. Kawai M, Kataoka YH, Sonobe J, et al. Non-surgical model for alveolar bone regeneration by bone morphogenetic protein-2/7 gene therapy. J Periodontol 2018;89:85–92.

28. Lektemur Alpan A, Kızıldağ A, Özdede M, et al. The effects of taxifolin on alveolar bone in experimental periodontitis in rats. Arch Oral Biol 2020;117:104823.

29. Perinetti G, Paolantonio M, Femminella B, et al. Gingival crevicular fluid alkaline phosphatase activity reflects periodontal healing/recurrent inflammation phases in chronic periodontitis patients. J Periodontol 2008;79(7):1200–7.

30. Al Swafeeri H, ElKenany W, Mowafy M, et al. Crevicular alkaline phosphatase activity during the application of two patterns of orthodontic forces. J Orthod 2015;42:5–13.

31. Pilawski I, Tulu US, Ticha P, et al. Interspecies comparison of alveolar bone biology, Part I: Morphology and physiology of pristine bone. JDR Clin Trans Res 2020;13. 2380084420936979.

32. Hlaing TT, Compston JE. Biochemical markers of bone turnover - uses and limitations. Ann Clin Biochem 2014;51:189–202.

33. Lee NK, Sowa H, Hinoi E, et al. Endocrine regulation of energy metabolism by the skeleton. Cell 2007;130:456–69.

34. Singh S, Kumar D, Lal AK. Serum osteocalcin as a diagnostic parameter for primary osteoporosis in women. J Clin Diagn Res 2015;9:RC04–7.

35. Garnero P, Vergnaud P, Hoyle N. Evaluation of a fully automated serum assay for total N-terminal propeptide of type I collagen in postmenopausal osteoporosis. Clin Chem 2008;54:188–96.

36. Gul SS, Griffiths GS, Stafford GP, et al. Investigation of a novel predictive biomarker profile for the outcome of periodontal treatment. J Periodontol 2017;88:1135–44.

37. Leppilahti JM, Sorsa T, Kallio MA, et al. The utility of gingival crevicular fluid matrix metalloproteinase-8 response patterns in prediction of site-level clinical treatment outcome. J Periodontol 2015;86:777–87.

38. Sculean A, Gruber R, Bosshardt DD. Soft tissue wound healing around teeth and dental implants. J Clin Periodontol 2014;41:S6–22.

39. Sexton WM, Lin Y, Kryscio RJ, et al. Salivary biomarkers of periodontal disease in response to treatment. J Clin Periodontol 2011;38:434–41.

40. Lee CH, Chen YW, Tu YK, et al. The potential of salivary biomarkers for predicting the sensitivity and monitoring the response to nonsurgical periodontal therapy: A preliminary assessment. J Periodontal Res 2018;53:545–54.

41. Gürsoy UK, Pussinen PJ, Salomaa V, et al. Cumulative use of salivary markers with an adaptive design improves detection of periodontal disease over fixed biomarker thresholds. Acta Odontol Scand 2018;76:493–6.

42. Pellegrini G, Rasperini G, Pagni G, et al. Local wound healing biomarkers for real-time assessment of periodontal regeneration: Pilot study. J Periodontal Res 2017;52:388–96.

43. Rakmanee T, Calciolari E, Olsen I, et al. Expression of growth mediators in the gingival crevicular fluid of patients with aggressive periodontitis undergoing periodontal surgery. Clin Oral Investig 2019;23:3307–18.

44. Taiete T, Monteiro MF, Casati MZ, et al. Local IL-10 level as a predictive factor in generalized aggressive periodontitis treatment response. Scand J Immunol 2019;90:e12816.

45. Koidou VP, Cavalli N, Hagi-Pavli E, et al. Expression of inflammatory biomarkers and growth factors in gingival crevicular fluid at different healing intervals following non-surgical periodontal treatment: A systematic review. J Periodontal Res 2020;55:801–9.

46. Caton J, Nyman S. Histometric evaluation of periodontal surgery. I. The modified Widman flap procedure. J Clin Periodontol 1980;7:212–23.

Moving?

Make sure your subscription moves with you!

To notify us of your new address, find your **Clinics Account Number** (located on your mailing label above your name), and contact customer service at:

Email: **journalscustomerservice-usa@elsevier.com**

800-654-2452 (subscribers in the U.S. & Canada)
314-447-8871 (subscribers outside of the U.S. & Canada)

Fax number: 314-447-8029

Elsevier Health Sciences Division
Subscription Customer Service
3251 Riverport Lane
Maryland Heights, MO 63043

*To ensure uninterrupted delivery of your subscription, please notify us at least 4 weeks in advance of move.

Printed and bound by CPI Group (UK) Ltd, Croydon, CR0 4YY

03/10/2024

01040404-0015